W9-BJG-925

WHEN THE TRIP CHANGES

A Traveler's Advisory to Colorectal Cancer

by Carol Larson

Illustrations by Rochelle Cunningham
Photos by Rodney Nelson

Carol Larson
15733 Randall Lane
Minnetonka, MN 55345

Original book designed by Donn Poll, Minnesota USA

Library of Congress catalog card number 0-9746008-0-6

Illustrations by Rochelle Cunningham
Photos by Rodney Nelson

When The Trip Changes
A Traveler's Advisory to Colorectal Cancer

For the many people and their families
who are facing colorectal cancer.

"Learning comes, but wisdom lingers"
–Alfred Lord Tennyson

Acknowledgments

I would never have come this far were it not for the encouragement of my brother, Red, when I was a youngster starting to write on my grandfather's typewriter in Sandstone, Minnesota. Red has been my chief editor and champion throughout my life.

I have a group of people to thank for reading and helping me make this book a reality: To Cookie, who has helped me to never, never face the fact that I might not be able to accomplish this project. You've always believed in what I could do.

To Paulette Bates Alden Writers' Group: Kathy Ogle, Barb Vaughan, Hazel Lutz, Amie Klempnauer, and Rita Benak. To the Minnetonka Writers' Group: Miles Canning, Mim Kagol, Suzy Lofquist, and Mike Wendle. Your guidance helped me through every chapter and every revision. To Jane Nielsen, Sandy Lyons, and husband, Dave , Norman and Judith Larson for all your wordsmithing and patience, helping me to revise the revisions.

To Rodney Nelson for your terrific photographs and inspiration. To Rochelle Cunningham for your delightful art work and your support. To Ruth Edstrom, Cindy Iverson, and Kristin Tabor for making my dreams come true. And finally, to Donn Poll and Brian Johnson who helped me bring my original manuscript to production, and Robert Anderson who labored over the artistry of bringing my pictures and graphics into focus. To Randy Johnson who patiently guided me through the technological process of this book. This book would not have gone into print without you!

There wouldn't be any book, of course, if I hadn't had the excellent medical care I was given to survive cancer. I especially want to thank Dr. Nemer, Dr. Finne, Dr. Sborov, Dr. Olsen, Dr. Tanghe, Dr.Immerman, and Dr. Rene. This list includes my nurses: Vicki and Julie, Michelle, Trish, and the nurses from Fairview Hospital, Edina, and Abbott Northwestern Hospital, Minneapolis. I also want to thank Mary Hughes for her guidance.

To my friends who have helped me live through harsh experiences without losing hope. Most of you have been mentioned in the book but I would not have survived as well as I did without you. I always knew you were there for me. To "Our Gang": Marilyn and Arnie Lubrecht, Noni Gillham, and our beloved departed friends, Joe Godava and John Olin. To the members of our gang who accompanied us to Italy: Pat and Dick

Myslajek and Rodney Nelson. To our tour leader, Guilia, and our traveling companion, Carolyn.

To Athena, Barb and Birdie, who have been my soul travelers, Dick and Judy, Mike and Kristine, Ron and Jaci, Lorice, our ever fun and supportive Scandinavian group, our high school and our neighborhood friends. To Penny, Marta, Barb, and Pat B. To Jennifer Elnicky for your support and making me look good while going through treatments. To the Minnetonka Library.

To my school chums Pam, Dave, Deb, Pam, Ina, and Carol, plus my coworkers Laura and Lidelle, friends from the staff, the secretaries, and administration of St. Louis Park High School, Bob Laney, Fran Crisman, and my very special students.

To all the suppers and years I shared with Mary Lou, Sandy, and Dee.

You all helped me through so many problems and gave me support when I needed it the most. Thank you, thank you, thank you.

To my sister and her family's endeavors to help me to remain a positive person.

And of course, my husband's and my family's efforts have been documented in these pages. To Dave, who took me to every doctor's appointment and stayed with me through every crisis. To my children Tami, Laura, and Jennifer whose lives were disrupted for more than a year, but who never complained about that fact. You inspired me to do my very best to get well. To Meg and Jean for being my guardian angels.

(Now I know why those Academy Award speeches go on so long.)

I'm sure I left people out, but you know who you are, and I thank you. I have been so blessed by wonderful people in my life!

Contents

Foreword

Many of you who have picked up this book have been diagnosed with colon or rectal cancer, know or love someone who has, or live in fear of it because of a family history of this illness. Some of you are interested in maintaining your health in whatever way you can. Others may simply be curious, looking for a good story, one that is true and honest. If you fall into one of these groups, you have opened the right book.

Colon and rectal cancer will affect an estimated 146,970 Americans in 2009, with slightly more cases occurring in women than in men. More than 49,920 men and women will die of this disease every year, most having lived with their cancer for a period of several years. It is the second most frequent cause of cancer death in men and women. Yet, despite these statistics, a conspiracy of secrecy is still attached to this illness. Despite our culture's ability to openly discuss many subjects once felt to be taboo, far too many of us feel that to speak of the intestine is somehow improper for polite company.

Carol Larson is courageous enough to ignore such rules. She faces the secrecy head on and stares it down. She helps us to understand, to laugh, and cry along with her as she describes her very individual but ultimately universal journey. Her experience as an educator — in an alternative program for teens, no less — serves her well in navigating difficult ground with skill, charm, insight and humor.

As a medical oncologist, I have counseled hundreds of patients with colon and rectal cancer as they face a multitude of decisions and find their way through today's bewildering medical system. Perhaps more than most other cancers, up-to-date treatment of colorectal cancer requires a multidisciplinary approach; that is, numerous medical doctors and professionals are involved at every step of the way. The team may require a general physician, a gastroenterologist, a general surgeon, a surgeon specializing in colorectal diseases, a medical oncologist, a radiation oncologist, an enterostomal therapist, oncology nurses skilled in delivering chemotherapy, and radiation oncology technicians and nurses.

Ms. Larson met all of these professionals, and more. I have rarely known someone who was able to describe her experience undergoing cancer treatment with such insight and intelligence. It is easy, in this day of the World Wide Web and online library research, to find factual information about illness and health. In fact, there is a flood of information available today, in nearly any hospital or library in the country; however, what is not so easy to come by is wisdom. Even as she was going through a difficult year of treatment, Carol was able to recognize that something else was happening to her: she was changing in ways she never imagined. Some changes led to grief and loss, but others resulted in dramatically positive benefits that spilled over to her family and friends.

When The Trip Changes: A Traveler's Advisory to Colorectal Cancer describes one woman's journey into hostile, foreign territory. It is territory I know well, and a land through which I have tried to guide many others. A guidebook is always a useful item to pack on a journey, and here is one of the best.

Kathleen Ogle, MD
Medical Oncologist

When The Trip Changes

A Traveler's Advisory
to Colorectal Cancer

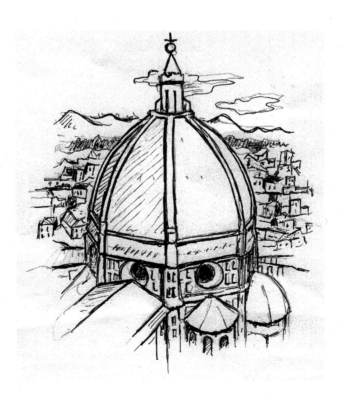

In memory of my Aunt Jean Dredge

This book is dedicated to the
doctors and nurses who
have given me such excellent care
and my husband, Dave, my family, and friends
who accompanied me on my journey
when my life was detoured by colorectal cancer.

With special thanks to my brother, Red,
a most groovy guy, who has given me,
and so many others, courage along the way…

Here's Looking at You, Kids

CHAPTER ONE

Facing the Unknown: Travel Preparations

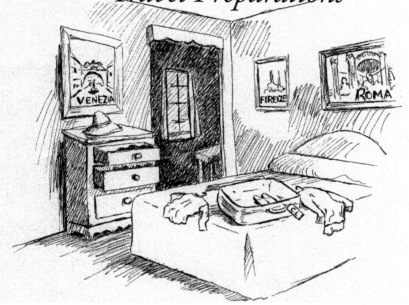

I'm leaving tomorrow to begin a tour of Italy! Even though it's the middle of May, I no longer have to wait until summer to travel, thanks to early retirement from my 24 years of teaching. After a harsh winter, my husband and three of our friends want to leave Minnesota and fly to warm, sunny places. My stacks of clothing are waiting to take a ride to Tuscan territory. I'm excited, but something is preventing me from packing. What's holding me back? I sit down by the empty suitcase on my bed and realize I'm folding in feelings of apprehension about this trip.

Coping with anxiety is nothing new for me anymore. Following a two-year struggle with colorectal cancer, misgivings are a regular occurrence for me, especially the psychological ones erected out of fear. I'm on the road to recovery, but I still feel vulnerable. Lingering aftereffects from my treatments have given me unusual problems from time to time and they are causing me doubts now. What if I need a hospital while we're in some small Italian town? Would they have the expertise to know what to do?

In the pocket of my suitcase I have carefully stored away names of Italian doctors and nurses in Rome who specialize in the care that I might need. My colorectal surgeon suggested if an emergency operation would be necessary, I could fly home immediately and the hospital staff here could take care of me.

"All of life is a risk," I have to remind myself.

I return to packing, choosing only clothes that will be the most useful. Even though our luggage will be taken care of during this 10-day bus tour, I want to travel light. Nevertheless, there has to be some room for frivolity too. I stuff clunky sandals into my carry-on bag. They might give me blisters if we walk very far, but still they do match my long, artsy olive skirt I'm bringing along. I'm having trouble fitting things in. It doesn't help that at the base of this bag, there is a plastic 9-by-12-inch container full of syringes and medical supplies for emergencies. The zipper to my carry-on bag doesn't quite close. I finally decide to toss out the sandals, along with some of my vanity, to give me more space.

What's happened is my ideas about travel, like my ideas about life, have been significantly altered. I used to plan my future like I was planning a trip, deciding on a destination, charting desired stop-offs, trying to follow a fixed itinerary. What I did not prepare for were the unexpected routes. Once diagnosed with cancer, regardless of my plans, I had to use all my navigating powers just to get my bearings.

Though cancer was hardly a blessing, there have been many valuable lessons that have come from that experience. While it's good to be reasonably cautious, fear can be immobilizing and make any journey more difficult than it has to be. Figuring out what's important determines the success of the journey. Clunky sandals, as cute as they are, don't count; traveling light does. Having a good guidebook and a map certainly helps. Still, I have learned that the only way to prepare for the future is to be open to change.

Warning Signs

When did I first know something was wrong? The awareness of potential danger began like a faint siren, hardly noticeable but demanding attention. My husband and I were driving to a party just two weeks before Christmas. The scene out the window reminded me of powdered sugar sprinkling onto white meringues. I thought to myself, Minnesota is a beautiful place to live. At that moment, I had an eerie revelation. I realized if I wanted to live in this world of magical seasons, I needed to check out some suspicious signs I had been ignoring. I turned to my husband, Dave.

"Could we stop at Urgent Care before we go to the party?"

"Now?" he said, perplexed. I rarely went to a doctor. "Are you sick?"

I had to think about it before I answered. "I'm not sure, but I might be."

I said nothing to him before that time indicating I was having any health problems, but I explained how tired I had been feeling and the minor spotting from my rectum I had noticed for almost a month. I just finished a grueling week at school (it's always grueling the week before a vacation, and my job as an alternative high school teacher was not an easy one). I tried to tell myself that the physical symptoms were just "natural" but some ancient wisdom inside of me was telling me this was not the case. I had been hoping the spotting was due to natural causes. It was bright red, and didn't that mean that it wasn't dangerous? Still, I knew this was something I hadn't experienced before and I could make no more excuses.

When the doctor at Urgent Care finally examined me, my worst fears were confirmed. His direct eye contact signaled he was serious about what he was going to say and this was not going to be an easy fix.

"Any kind of unexplained bleeding is a red flag. You need to call your doctor right away Monday morning and schedule a colonoscopy. Don't let them lose any time getting you in."

As we walked out to the car, the cold air seemed to cut deep and matched our concerns.

"Do you want to go home?" Dave asked.

I thought about it briefly. We needed to be among friends, sharing the warmth of a fire and some good conversation. I replied, "I think we should go to the party."

Dave and I grew up in the same neighborhood and reunite with people we knew from high school at this time every year. We both looked forward to this event. I continued to say, "We probably could use some distraction." He nodded in agreement.

The next morning, I went to the phone book to call "my" doctor and was puzzled about whom to call. I had rarely been sick, and only went in to have a yearly physical with my gynecologist. I had no "primary" doctor, so to speak, so I called my gynecologist and he referred me to a gastroenterologist.

I found that I didn't have to contend with him putting me off. Within a few days I was scheduled for a colonoscopy.

Security Check-in — The Colonoscopy

Sometimes a person goes in for a preliminary exam in a doctor's office called a sigmoidoscopy and then, if a problem is detected, a colonoscopy is ordered. In my case, because of the bleeding and tiredness, my doctors decided that I should go straight to the colonoscopy.

I knew very little about my colon. Who does? It was like my using the plumbing in our house without having the foggiest notion of what to do if the pipes became faulty. I consulted a medical book to find out the basics: The colon is your large intestine or large bowel. It is approximately three inches in diameter and five to six feet long. Its job is to absorb water and work like a trash compactor, forming waste matter that can be eliminated through the anus.

Specifically, rectal cancers are found in the last six inches of the digestive tract, and colon cancers are above the rectum but both rectal and colon cancers are commonly called "colorectal cancers." Colorectal cancers develop slowly over the years in the lower portions of the digestive tract and if discovered early enough can be eliminated through surgery. Most colorectal cancers begin with polyps, a flat or grape-like growth that can be detected through a colonoscopy, or a sigmoidscope.

The advantage of a colonoscopy is that it will enable the doctor to see the entire colon. It's usually done on an outpatient basis in a hospital. If a polyp is discovered, it can be removed painlessly and examined microscopically to determine any malignancy. Doctors differ on what kind of preparation for a colonoscopy they want you to take. I wasn't aware that I could request any alternatives.

This particular gastroenterologist wanted me to ingest the kind of solution that would be mixed with a gallon of cold water. My directions were to drink an 8 oz. glass of this liquid every 10 minutes the night before the test.

It sounded easy enough, but when I looked at how much water I was going to have to swallow, I had imagined myself filling up like a water balloon. I did not have to worry about that predicament. After three glasses, the water did not stay in me for any length of time. It was called "Golytely" which is a misnomer if there ever was one. I did not go lightly between running to the bathroom, shuddering as I downed each glass of the substance, and shivering with cold as the water flushed through me. I was told to drink the Golytely cold, as it was supposed to "taste" better this way. Perhaps. I learned later that there is an alternative two-glass version of this preparation, which is much, much easier to endure.

Regardless, I followed all directions and put discomfort behind me, so to speak, checking into the hospital the next morning fully cleansed, like the spirit of a true Minnesotan, having made an Olympic effort to brave the elements.

In contrast, the colonoscopy was easy. A soothing nurse sat by me while I lay on a cart waiting for the test.

"Don't worry," she assured me. "The test is much easier to take than the preparation."

The anesthesia injected in my arm relaxed me, a warm blanket comforted me, and the gastroenterologist lulled me with his kind voice through the whole procedure. Two polyps were discovered and removed painlessly. The doctor said they looked benign, but they needed to make sure with a biopsy. He promised to call me when he got the test results back, and I was sent home with optimism.

In fact, I was so relieved, that I didn't even consider in the following week how much I was tying up our phones by being on the Internet, creating lessons I could use with our students after vacation. As I was preparing food and dressing up for our family Christmas Eve party, I got a call from the gastroenterologist who had done the colonoscopy. The fact that he should be calling me on December 24th filled me with apprehension.

"Mrs. Larson, I'm sorry to call you on this day, but I've been trying to get in touch with you for the last two days and I really need to give you this news." His voice was apologetic, but insistent. "One of the polyps we biopsied turned out to be malignant."

I was stunned. I felt blindsided from behind.

"I'm pretty sure we got it all in surgery during the colonoscopy, but I suggest that you call up a colorectal surgeon immediately."

He gave me his recommendation of a doctor to contact, and then I hung up the phone. Before I could collect my thoughts, the phone rang again. As if by ESP, my friend Cookie from California called. As soon as she heard my voice, she asked, "Carol, are you all right?"

I blurted out what the doctor had said. That was the first time that I spoke the word "cancer." Just like I had the wind knocked out of me, I was gasping for air. We both cried. I told her I had to get off the phone so we could go on with the day.

The concerns of the moment took precedent over my worries. It was Christmas, a blessed time in our family's life, and I didn't want to have one minute of it spoiled. I decided to keep the doctor's diagnosis to myself. It could be shared later. I repeated the doctor's assurances like a drug, over and over, trying to anesthetize myself from the effect of the news. I shoved the conversation I had with the doctor in the background so the healthy part of me could celebrate the good things in life.

Miraculously, we had one of our best Christmases ever, although it seems we always say that each year as we become more attached to our expanding family. Jenny, our youngest daughter, had graduated from college and had started a new job. Our middle daughter, Laura, was engaged to Scott, and we were making plans for their wedding in July. Our oldest daughter, Tami, and her husband, Dean, had adopted a daughter, Courtney, now three-and-a-half years old, who was adding another dimension of love to our lives. My sister, Beverly, and her family lived in California, but my older brother, Red lived nearby. His wife, Sandy, their three children, plus their families, make up a fun and endearing group.

I finally told Red, Sandy, and my daughters later in the week. People have to deal with this problem in their own way, but I found it easier for me to break the news individually on the phone, as a way to give us more time to get used to the fact I had cancer and to adjust to that fact. For us, it was a wake-up call. Life was not something we could take for granted, no matter what age you are. One thing was certain. There was no way now to pretend this wasn't really happening. My diagnosis was out in the open and we had to move on to the next step of how to deal with the reality.

Obstacles to Good Health

Faced with this situation, I asked myself, how did I get on this road in the first place? Was there something I did that "gave" me cancer?

I eventually learned no one knows exactly what makes someone susceptible to colorectal cancer, but there are some risk factors: a diet high in fat and low in fruits and vegetables; a sedentary life style; people with inflammatory bowel diseases; people with family histories of colon cancer. In my case, the only real risk factors that applied were my family history. Many of my relatives have had cancer, although we also have a fair number of cancer survivors too.

I've had suggestions from well-meaning friends in the past about lessening the stress in my life. For 24 years I was a teacher working in specific programs consisting of students struggling with high school. It was not an easy job, but I loved it, and I cared very much for my students. I always felt I rolled with the punches and handled stress well, but it was difficult work, nevertheless. About ten years ago, my husband lost his job due to corporate downsizing and the ramifications of that event certainly added to the stress in our house. He eventually got another interesting job working for a non-profit social service organization, but there were tough times in between. I would be the last to say that my life has not had its strains; however, as I look around me, there are other people who I know have significant problems too, many dealing with far greater tensions than I've had to face.

It does not seem to follow factually that a stressful life "gives" people cancer. What might be true is that stress lowers the resistance of people fighting off any disease and this certainly could be the case as far as cancer was concerned.

Probably the key factor in my situation was that I should have had a colonoscopy examination before I got into any trouble. I don't remember being aware that this was something everyone over age fifty should do, or anyone else at risk or showing signs of trouble. I think there's a reason I was not well informed. I thought of colorectal cancer as a man's disease, not realizing that almost half of the people diagnosed are women. I didn't know that fact, because as a general rule, people didn't talk about colorectal cancer. Unfortunately, this very silence contributes to the sad fact that we as a nation do not take enough precautions to prevent this disease by getting appropriate screening.

Colorectal cancer is the second most common cancer causing death in the United States today, but it can be prevented and is highly treatable if caught in time. If my doctors had waited to give me a colonoscopy after my visit to Urgent Care, I might not be alive today. That's why I feel so strongly that we need to break the taboos about discussing it and raise the awareness of the public so that lives are not lost needlessly out of ignorance and fear.

I started out vowing I would only tell a select few about my diagnosis. As my journey progressed, I reversed this decision and turned it into a personal mission to bring this disease into the open. I now find myself sharing some things I thought I would never tell another soul. There were invaluable lessons I learned as I became an experienced traveler in the journey of regaining my health. I can only hope passing on these lessons will make it easier for those diagnosed with colorectal cancer to take better care of their health and to be less afraid. It's not the end of the road. The path may be rocky at times, but there will be respites and new perspectives gained along the way.

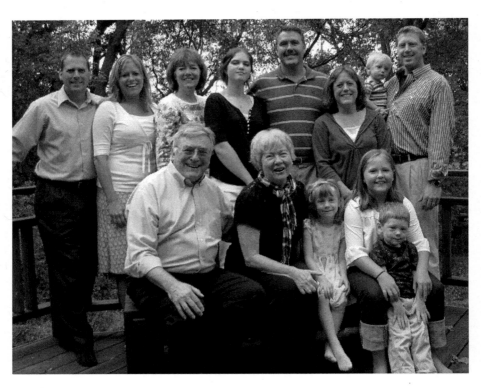

Our family 2009

**Tips for Travelers Who May Be Facing Colorectal Cancer:

- Listen to your instincts and don't let any embarrassment you might feel prevent you from going for a checkup.
- Regardless of the slight discomfort you may have to endure during tests, it's worth it to stop cancer at its earliest stages.
- Pay attention to any unexplained bleeding. Only an accurate examination by a doctor can determine the true cause.
- Other warning signals may be vague and hard to notice. There might be bloating, changes in bowel habits, or minor fatigue. All of those symptoms might be indicative of some other problem, but they need to be immediately checked out for cancer.
- Talk to someone you trust about the fears you may be having.
- The beginning of this journey may turn out to be the loneliest part of your trip until you can connect with caregivers or other cancer survivors. This would be an ideal time to attend some cancer workshops or join a support group.
- To learn more about guidelines for screening, contact the website www.preventcancer.org/colorectal.

Dave & Carol

Chian

John

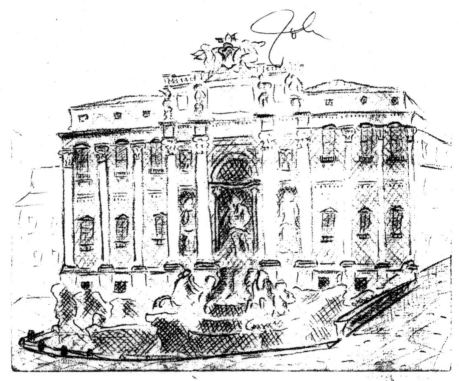

CHAPTER TWO

Gathering information: "When in Rome…"

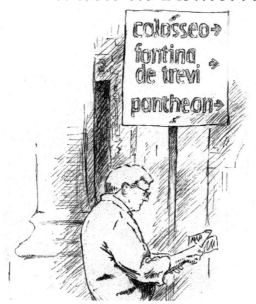

When we first arrive in Italy I feel like Dorothy, landing in Oz and commenting to her dog, "Toto, I don't think we're in Kansas anymore." We are definitely in a different culture. Almost everyone around us is speaking Italian. Even though we know a few catch phrases and words, we have to keep consulting our dictionaries to translate. "Ciao" is not a request for food…

From the airport, we follow our leader, an attractive blonde named Giulia, to the hotel. Once there, she efficiently takes charge of our most immediate needs. We won't be able to get our rooms until later in the day, so we decide to explore our neighborhood, which is walking distance away from ancient Rome. We consult our maps and follow a path to the Pantheon, the Spanish Steps, and the Trevi Fountain. This section of Rome is an artist's delight of a modern city mixed in with buildings looking like they were made of clay. Churches resemble ornate pottery. Between burnt tones of salmon and mustard, beige is the dominant color.

One of our friends comments, "It's very old" and we laugh, because it is so true. There is a different scale of measuring history here. In America, buildings constructed merely 150 years ago are considered landmarks. In Italy, that's just a bat of an eyelash.

We become immediately aware of the raucous sounds of the city. Italy is noisy! Horns are honking, small putt-putt motors are spurting fumes, and people are talking to each other louder with great intensity. There is a rhythm to conversations blending in with a background of traffic jazz.

Although somewhat intimidated, we want to fit into this environment. We want to know at least enough Italian to get by. We want to be able to understand how to cross the street without getting hit. Why aren't there more accidents? The whistle of the traffic patrolman, neatly dressed almost like a naval officer, seems to be blowing all the time. Young, attractive women whiz by on motorcycles wearing fashionable leather jackets and helmets. Signals are working, but no one seems to follow them. It looks to us like the pushiest driver wins.

Back at our hotel, Guilia gathers us together to explain how things work around here, and what paths to avoid. She gives us an itinerary, but already things have changed since we started making our plans, and there are side trips to allow us to go other places if we want to. Feeling confused and unsure of ourselves, we move closer together, content to stick to our own little group of five. It doesn't take us too long, however, to start to get to know the other passengers. By the time we go to dinner, we have acquired another companion, a woman named Carolyn from New York. After studying the information Guilia gave us, we plan our itinerary and feel much more confident about where we will be going.

That was our initiation to Rome, but it is a predictable pattern when finding your way in any unfamiliar environment. When I first entered the world of dealing with cancer, I needed to learn new phrases and vocabulary in order to become more fluent; doctors and nurses became my tour guides; finding my way around hospitals and doctors' offices was a challenge; new routines had to be followed and I had to discover ways to get around.

I wanted to stick just to the people I knew, but gradually I had to learn to trust others. I found I had to continually gather information. There is a learning curve with cancer that goes way up when you are diagnosed. Just like in Rome, I needed to educate myself as quickly as I could. It was all about getting acclimated.

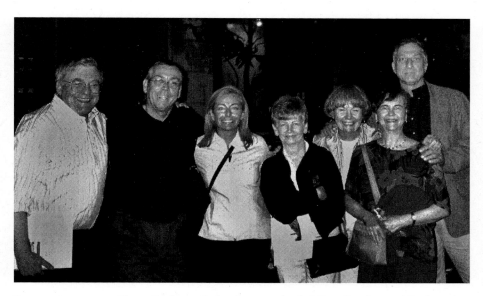

Beginning our tour: Dave, Rodney, Guila, (our tour leader) Pat, Carolyn and Dick with me at the bus.

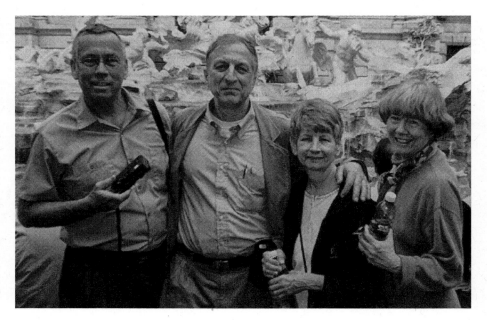

Our first day in Rome by the Trevi Fountain.

Initiation — Stage One

We have a core of mostly high school friends that have been together so long, we're like family. I think of them like characters out of an "Our Gang" comedy. The day after Christmas, six of us from that group rented a townhouse in northern Minnesota to go cross-country skiing. I debated about marring our vacation telling them about my diagnosis, but I had to do it. It would be too difficult calling long distance to schedule my doctor's appointment without them knowing about it. So, when we were gathered in the kitchen, I solemnly declared, "I've got something I have to tell you."

It was as if someone pushed the pause button on the VCR. All action stopped while I told them I had cancer. I repeated the doctor's statement that probably he got it all, and that the sample from the polyps looked like the cancer was self-contained. Nevertheless, it was necessary for me to make an appointment right away with a colorectal surgeon in Minneapolis.

It was a dramatic moment downplayed by the fact none of us wanted to overreact.

This was the first time an illness threatened our future together and it was a sobering disclosure. I made my first call, long-distance, to the colorectal surgeon's office. As it happens with cancer patients, I was given an appointment promptly, as soon as I returned from winter break. We finished the week acting as normal as possible, but we were aware that we had entered another world, foreign to all of us.

More unexpected news awaited me the following week when I went back to school. Ironically, the two people who I teamed with were dealing with people in their respective families having significant health problems. Then I told them about my situation. We looked at each other in disbelief. Wasn't it just supposed to be a superstition about bad luck running in threes? Apprehensively, we started the New Year. It was a reminder that even though I was coping with my fears of cancer, life goes on. Other people have problems too.

Sight-seeing with a Purpose: The Flexible Sigmoidscope

Three days later, I had my first appointment with a colorectal surgeon. Nervous as I was, I was relieved to learn later that meeting with a surgeon does not mean you are automatically going to have an operation.

This is a doctor who is an expert in the surgical and non-surgical treatment of colon and rectal problems. I asked my brother and my husband to come with me on my first appointments when there were major consultations involved. That turned out to be a wise thing to do. Aside from it being an added source of support, it was helpful to me to have them listen to the same information I was receiving. I needed to have a clear message about what the doctor was saying and it was hard to keep my emotions from interfering with my ability to listen. I took along a small notebook, writing down specific words that could be looked up in a dictionary later.

We first met in the colorectal surgeon's office, not an examination room. The doctor had a dramatic presence and a distinctive voice. Completely in his domain, he inspired confidence. We were given a clear-cut explanation of the situation and why he was authorizing a sigmoidscope. He drew us a picture of where the polyps were found, and what had been taken out during the biopsy.

"Kind of like the divot a golfer might make on a golf course," he explained.

At this point, he was predicting that the gastroenterologist had removed all of the cancer with the polyp; the cancer had been enclosed and contained.

"Cancer is measured according to stages. If all your tests are good, you will be considered to be in Stage One."

I interjected, "And that means...?"

"Statistically, your chances are 90% for survival. We do nothing else except watch and wait to see if it changes."

Hopeful, I went into another room to have my sigmoidscope examination.

The last part of the colon is S-shaped and is called "the sigmoid colon." Using a lighted tube, called a "sigmoidscope", the doctor examined 30 inches of my lower colon and rectum. By pumping air into the tube, he was able see the lining of the colon as well. The entire test took less than ten minutes. I felt some minor cramping, not unlike just before a bowel movement.

I found that deep breathing and relaxation exercises helped me "relax", although admittedly, it's hard to relax with a foreign instrument probing your subterranean interior. I also found it helpful to count out the seconds of the most uncomfortable part. Still, the payoffs for such an exam far outweigh any discomfort a person might experience. This test reveals up to 70% of all polyps in the colon. The preparation, in my case, was much simpler and less uncomfortable compared to the colonoscopy. I was required to take two prepared Fleet enemas, two hours before the examination.

After the exam, we came back to his office to talk. Rather than rushing us along, he listened to our questions and took the time to explain what he saw. He delivered some welcome news.

"I could find no visual signs of polyps or cancer," he concluded. "I'm fairly certain the gastroenterologist removed any malignancy during the colonoscopy."

"Even so," he promised, "We're going to watch you like a hawk."

He finished by suggesting I make another appointment with one of his associates for a rectal ultrasound.

"Just to make sure," he added.

Video Travelogue —The Ultrasound

To determine that I really was in Stage One, I needed to have an ultrasound examination. Again, I was given an appointment right away, which was a clear message of urgency. The following week I was scheduled for the test in Abbott Hospital, connected to The Virginia Piper Institute in Minneapolis, which has a prestigious reputation as a cancer research center. As I walked through the door, the significance of where I was hit me. I clutched my coat around me like a warm quilt shielding me from the draft of fear I was experiencing.

This time, when I arrived at the doctor's office, an amiable nurse interviewed me and escorted me into an examining room where I undressed and lay on my side in a fetal position waiting for test to begin. Another nurse talked to me about the procedure. When the doctor came into the room, he immediately put me more at ease by his folksy, affable style. Still, the concern in his voice was unmistakable.

During the rectal ultrasound, a long flexible tube is inserted into the rectum. High frequency sound waves produced images, which we watched on a television-like screen.

I found the whole ordeal was again tolerable by using deep breathing to relax myself, and also because the pictures we were seeing were rather fascinating. It reminded me of the 50's when we used to watch TV test patterns for the very first time, attentively looking for an image in the scanning fields. This was more suspenseful, however. Whatever he was searching for, I didn't want him to find.

As the test progressed, I grew concerned with how long it was taking. When it was all over, he frowned and said, "I'm not too satisfied with the picture. Maybe because it hasn't been that long since you had the polyps removed, but the results are too fuzzy for me to see much of anything and I don't like that." He paused.

"If it were up to me, I would prefer to cut out the questionable part of your colon (a resection) and look at it under a microscope, but that might be overkill."

This was alarming to me. A resection would be major surgery.

"I'll call your colorectal surgeon tomorrow about waiting for a month until I can get a clearer picture. He'll call you later in the day."

He also had the thankless job of informing me if he did see more acute signs of cancer in the second ultrasound, I would have to have radiation and chemotherapy as part of my treatment, along with the resection of my colon.

My thoughts went racing ahead of the words he was uttering. As nice as he was, I resisted what he was saying and tried to discard what I heard once I left his office.

The message stayed with me, however. During that night I woke up and replayed the doctor's speech over and over again in my mind. I tried to apply reason to the situation. Surely I couldn't be in much danger. I had sought help within a month of the first signs that I might be in trouble. I never had trouble with my digestive system before. I did all the "right" things, like eating lots of fiber, fruit and vegetables. I prayed in my own way of praying for solace while I was waiting to find out what the doctors would decide to do.

The next morning I reached into my jewelry box and slipped on a Claddaugh ring that Cookie sent me in January. Being Irish, I believed in its magic of promising good luck to the one who was wearing the silver band around their finger. I kept twisting it in circles the following day while I was at work and marveled at how well I was managing my anxiety.

Later in the afternoon I realized how upset I had been. Instead of going directly home, I drove aimlessly around for almost an hour, completely lost on the road, absorbed with the dread of what the doctors might say. When I arrived home, Dave told me the colorectal surgeon had called with some good news.

"The doctor said he's not the least bit worried," he reported. "He's sure the swelling was due to surgery, and to come back in about a month for a second ultrasound just to be on the safe side."

I think now that perhaps the doctor's message might not have been that optimistic, but rather that Dave was doing some of his own interpreting. It didn't matter. It was what I wanted to believe too. I wanted to resume my safe routines without venturing further into the world of disease.

Finding a Good Doctor

This was the beginning of a path that would involve many detours.

A good doctor, like an experienced tour guide, can direct you to the right locations and help you form a superior itinerary. Most doctors try to perform these services but the constraints on their time may be prohibitive.

Before I was diagnosed with cancer, I must admit, I was frequently annoyed with the system, having to wait six weeks for an appointment and occasionally trying to put pressure on the receptionist to "squeeze me in." My attitude has changed. Now the first thing I tell the receptionist for a normal checkup is that the reason I am calling is not an emergency, if that is the case. I have learned that very sick people are filling up those slots of time. At least, this is true of a doctor dealing with cancer patients.

When I entered into a new category of being a cancer patient, I discovered I was also given top level care. I happened to be lucky to be referred to professionals that suited me well. Other people I have talked to have not been so lucky, and years later are still lamenting they should have switched at the very beginning.

In working with doctors and nurses I came up with my own list of "C-Rations" that I needed in my health care providers:

- Competency
- Conscientiousness
- Communication
- Concern
- Compatibility

Learning the Language of "Medicine Land"

The quickest way I found out what doctors, nurses, or technicians were saying was to simply ask them. Medical terminology sometimes sounds like a foreign language, and there were times I even had to ask them to write down the words or pronounce them. This isn't a needless exercise. It became important to specifically be able to tell other caregivers what test, medication, or procedure I had been given.

Sometimes words would be said to me that I knew before, like "benign" meaning good and "malignant" meaning bad, but it seemed Doublethink to call a bad test "positive" and a good test "negative." That's the way it works, though.

Just like trying to speak a foreign language, however, I found I could overcome my lack of understanding by the tone of my voice and a certain measure of consideration.

One thing I learned from the start: Always, always be as nice to the receptionists as you can be. First of all, they're overworked; secondly they have power! It doesn't make any more sense to tell a receptionist off than it does to scold a traffic cop. With both, being unpleasant gives you diminishing returns.

Passports — Keeping Good Records

As my care became more complex, I learned to keep proper records if I was going to submit any forms to insurance companies and be able to easily access this information.

Important Records to keep:
- Health insurance policies and resources
- Health insurance and/or Medicare numbers
- Phone numbers and addresses of doctors, clinics, and hospitals
- Phone numbers and addresses of local pharmacies

I stored other health related data I kept in a folder at home in a fireproof place with specific dates and procedures including prescriptions and dosages, phone calls, and a log of conversations written down. I also included records of past significant medical history, lists of all medications currently being taken, lists of allergies, and a copy of a Health Care Directive.

**Tips for Travelers Diagnosed With Colorectal Cancer

- Gather all the information that you can as soon as you find out about your diagnosis.
- Be selective when choosing a doctor. As a new traveler in this territory, remember: you have a right to choose a doctor that you feel is the best for your situation. This may mean that, after meeting with one doctor, you will want to go to another for a second opinion. It's also important to select someone that you feel comfortable with on a personal level. Good guides can make a huge difference in the quality of your trip.
- Take along another person when consulting the doctor and ask them to take notes. You can look up the words or the definitions later.
- Keep all of your records in one place, like in a drawer or a file. Note all of your appointments on a calendar, according to time, doctor, and procedure.

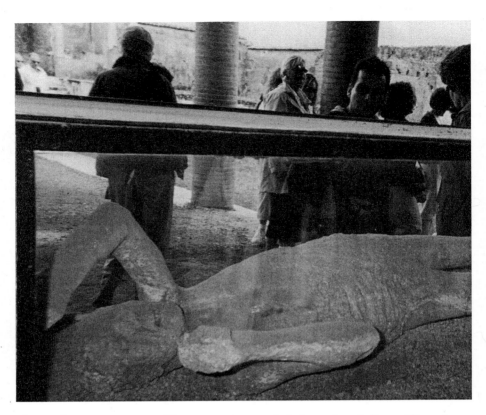

Plaster of Paris impressions of Pompeii victims reminded me of my feelings of fear when my diagnosis of cancer became more advanced.

CHAPTER THREE

Potential Dangers:
Pompeii

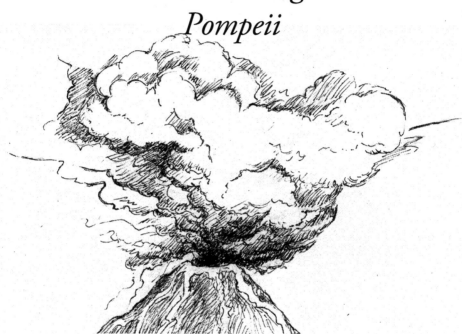

O ur first destination on this tour, Pompeii, reminds us that sometimes life can change within moments. On a summer morning in
AD 79, the earth's crust shifted, a volcano erupted, and lives became
endangered. Molten rock flowed from nearby Mount Vesuvius.

A gigantic cloud rose like an angry god spewing smoke. The sky turned
pitch black with hot ashes and pumice plunging down on the unsuspecting
inhabitants below. Given their lack of scientific knowledge, perhaps people
thought that "Charun," Etruscan god of the underworld, was expressing his
wrath. Perhaps that thought made some of the people cringe and hide in the
corners of their houses. Through the day, the burning hot coals built up to a
height of twelve feet. Most of the 10,000 people escaped, but about 2,000
were doomed to a hellish death by the suffocating heat. The world would not
know what occurred at Pompeii if it weren't for an enterprising archaeologist
who in 1860 uncovered most of its horrific secrets. Now, as we are guided
through the ruins, a question crosses my mind: why did some people take
action and some remain behind?

We follow a path through the ruins of this ghost town. As I look at their artifacts, mosaics, and courtyards, I am surprised at the sophistication of these ancient people. It has been interesting and rather eerie, but I am a tourist totally removed from the catastrophe until we turn the corner and I come face to face with the terror of that day. When we walk into one of the preserved courtyards, I am suddenly overcome by a feeling of "déjà vu."

We are looking at the plaster of Paris body casts, impressions of the victims of Pompeii entombed in glass. It is panic preserved in motion. Bodies unable to escape the worst torments of the mind. The writhing replicas of anguish arouse something familiar in me.

An agonized cry seems to resonate from these gray and silent replicas. Dread. Fear. The connection is that I remember experiencing these emotions when my diagnosis changed, although I never fully expressed them to anyone. As the tour guide drones on, I also know now why some people ran away, and some stayed. It is that moment of truth, that "momento de verite." The anxiety becomes crippling. There is a transient moment of time when, in spite of your fears, if you don't act quickly, you may be forever petrified in stone.

Unexpected Perils — The Second Diagnosis

After my first ultrasound I threw myself into a month of schoolwork while waiting for my second test. At times I even forgot the cancer and focused on creating curriculum, over which I had some degree of control. My coworkers' family members were overcoming their health problems and they were relieved. Our students worked hard trying to pass their graduation standards test, and we, their teachers, were proud of them. It was on the crest of these good feelings that I went in for my second examination.

The procedure went the same as before. While the doctor was probing my rectum with an endoscope, we were both looking at the sound waves on the screen. He was talking pleasantly to me, trying to help me relax. I learned during my first test that the white dots were benign, being less dense, but black dots were ominous. What I was staring at alarmed me.

My attention was fixed on three dreaded dark invaders. The room became very quiet. The lighthearted kidding ended. The only sound was the beeping of the machine announcing the bad news. The doctor's silence told me he was reluctant to broadcast the results. When he started to plot quadrants over them, I succumbed to despair. My body stiffened. In a sympathetic, soft voice, he said, "I'm sorry. It looks like the cancer has spread to your lymph nodes."

There I was, writhing in fear, like those stone bodies of Pompeii. I curled up, not moving. My heart was racing from adrenaline running through my veins.

"I have to cut off a little of each node to have it biopsied," he apologized. "This isn't going to be easy. Hang on."

His snipping didn't hurt, really. Maybe I was just numb, but I wasn't feeling any physical pain as he went through the business of removing each piece from my rectum. I lay there, filled with dread as we discussed my future.

"As I told you before, if the tests came out positive, you're going to need a resection, radiation, and chemotherapy."

I held back tears, grimacing like one of those plaster of Paris casts encased in glass. I tried to respond, to organize my thoughts, my life by groping for the familiar, the old routines I desperately wanted to use to protect me.

"B…but I can't take off time at this point. I'm really needed at school."

My voice was a shaky plea for more time. I wanted to deny the hot, molten mortal feelings erupting in my mind.

"And my daughter, Laura. I have to help plan her wedding. She's getting married in five months."

He wasn't buying any of it. Solemnly he said, "You need to take care of your health first, you know."

I knew what he was saying made sense. I knew that my life had taken a momentous turn. I knew that to deny the danger would be the worst course of action I could take.

It seems trivial now, but the first question I asked was, "Will I lose my hair?" The thought of losing my hair was excruciating. I couldn't think beyond that question to ask any others that might involve more serious issues.

"Probably not." he responded, "Not with the chemo you take for this kind of cancer, but an oncologist will be able to tell you more."

An oncologist. I was going to have to see an oncologist. Words like "chemo," "radiation" and "resection" kept echoing through my mind.

He finished, I dressed, and Dave came into the room. He looked disbelieving as the doctor repeated the news.

"Is it for sure the lymph nodes are malignant?" I asked, pleading for a way out.

"I'd stake my reputation on it," he answered. "The biopsy will tell us for sure."

I found myself fighting facts. I walked out, desperately hoping, in spite of what we saw on that screen, the black dots would turn out benign. After all, I had close calls before with questionable mammograms.

I spent the next two days in suspended belief waiting for the final results to come in. I knew I was in deep trouble, but I wasn't going to accept that fact until I actually knew for sure. Waiting in itself is a kind of litmus test for one's ability to withstand anxiety. It is, in some ways, worse than the actual ordeal. More than anything else, I wanted the waiting to be over.

At 9:00 a.m. as I was in front of my class, the phone rang. I told the students to begin to fill out their worksheets as I answered the call. It was from my doctor who had done the ultrasound. He asked, "Is this a good time to talk?" I should have replied, "No" but I was too anxious to wait any longer.

"I'm sorry to tell you this, but we got the results back on your ultrasound, and the cancer has metastasized to some of the adjacent lymph nodes, so we're going to have to begin a program of radiation and chemotherapy immediately and then schedule you for a resection."

Cancer had spread to my lymph nodes. He would call my colorectal surgeon immediately. I weakly replied I understood what he was saying. He ended the conversation by telling me with conviction, "I want you to know we're going to fight this."

I hung up the phone and faced the truth. The good health I had taken for granted had broken down. My life was rerouted on a momentous detour. I had to get major repairs in order to survive. As I was noticeably shaken, my coworkers took over my class arranging with my principal for me to leave for the day. I got into my coat and drove home, wanting to get to a place of safety. Dave was at a conference, so I called my brother, Red. He told me he'd be right over and we'd go for a ride.

At a moment like this, when the itinerary changes in your life, you need a champion, someone who will help you with the heavy burdens of life and who will lead you to a place of refuge. In the past, my brother took on this role for me. This time was no different.

When Red came in the front door, I blurted out the message from the doctor. He was consoling as we left our house. We decided to drive to Waverly, a small town in Minnesota about an hour away where our uncle Homer once lived, mostly because it provided us with a destination. I was crying and talking a lot, and my brother let me do that. We talked about cancer, about how it had affected our whole family, how my dad overcame it when he was 50 and lived to 85, how my aunt overcame it and lived until she was 98. It was entirely possible that I could survive it as well. Rationality entered the picture and I started to settle down.

In our genetic pool, overcoming cancer was a logical outcome. We kept on driving until we came to Montrose and found a place to eat that was called, unbelievably, "Red's Café." It seemed like the perfect spot at this particular time. I ordered eggs and bacon, my favorite comfort food, and weirdly enough, I was actually laughing at some of Red's jokes (I must have been sick) and having a good time. How could this be? I had cancer that had metastasized into my lymph nodes. I was going to have to face some aggressive measures if I was going to live. I wasn't denying this fact anymore. And yet, there we were, enjoying each other's company, talking about family things.

When he brought me home, I was feeling much more secure. My principal phoned encouraging me to take some time off from school to adjust to the news. I finally reached David by phone, and we made plans to go up to the North Shore for the weekend.

Later in the afternoon, friends from school dropped by when they heard the news; one, with a chocolate Easter bunny, one with some french fries from McDonald's (our favorite splurge) and one retired pal who offered to come in and take over my class if I needed a substitute. Small, huge gifts reminding me of the good times we had shared together. Little by little, the diagnosis started to lose its tremendous power to suffocate me with its heat. I called school and told them I was taking off on Friday until Tuesday.

Our daughters Tami, Laura, and Jennifer came over that night. In a way, the previous waiting had some beneficial aspects to it, but you never really can prepare for this kind of news. From that standpoint, we had one of our finest moments as a family. They let me know we would all pull together. I wouldn't have to fight this battle without support. I tried to assure them as much as I could that eventually everything would be all right. We took the calendar out and counted up the days until Laura would be getting married. There would probably be plenty of time for recovery from surgery before she walked down that aisle. I needed more information about how my treatments would be scheduled, but we started plotting ways in which we could work around them. I needed to sit and talk with the girls in the living room, so Dave took care of phone calls coming in from concerned friends. Sarge, Jenny's black lab, sat with his head in my lap. All of this helped. Oh, how it helped!

Points of Departure — Coping With a New Diagnosis

The next day, Dave and I drove up to the North Shore of Lake Superior, about 25 miles from the Canadian border. This was early March and it was still quite cold, but our room had a huge picture window overlooking the water.

As a child, visiting the North Shore was a yearly summer ritual for our family. I learned to love its rugged coastline as part of my heritage. The next morning, when I awoke, I knew why I chose to come up to this location. Here I was closer to my faith in God and my own particular spiritual beliefs than in any other place. The lake extended to a distance that blended in with the sky, with tinsels of sunlight sparkling on the water like promises of a better day. Up here, I knew I could find the confidence to solve any problem that needed to be solved.

Whenever I am troubled, I start writing in my journal randomly, and without censorship, as a way to clarify my thoughts. My fears transferred unto a written page:

"I am so afraid. What harsh news. I can't settle down, even though I'm looking upon waves that should be soothing to my soul. Everything I see is colored by the news that I received yesterday from the doctor. Every aspect of my life is going to change, and oh, I don't want that to happen. Some things I never wanted to change…"

"Am I fearing death? Don't think so. Not at this point in time. But I am afraid of the future. Of pain. Of the unknown. I have to remember some good could come out of this experience too. That's the way life works…I think I am afraid of being afraid. What am I going to have to face?"

What became clear to me was that I needed more information. I was scheduled to meet with my colorectal surgeon right after the weekend but I didn't know enough at this point to even ask the right questions. This would be my first line of attack, I reasoned, so I spent the rest of the morning reading all I could on colorectal cancer.

That was how I confronted the situation. However, Dave has an opposite way of dealing with the anxiety. He was struggling with all the recent happenings and had been significantly sleep-deprived the last few days. While I obsessively searched for information, he slept. When we finally started to talk in the afternoon about how we were going to spend the next few months, he wasn't convinced that I had heard the doctor correctly, and that it just couldn't be as bad as I imagined. Didn't I, after all, go in to see the doctor almost immediately when I first started to spot? Didn't the doctor tell us on our first consultation that I would be put on only a watchful schedule of tests? Maybe the colorectal surgeon wouldn't agree with what the other doctor was saying. Maybe the ultrasound wasn't all that accurate.

This conversation was maddening to me. I wanted to adopt Dave's version of the dilemma, but I needed to face reality. I was preparing my battles, and he was telling me there wasn't a war. When I proposed I could probably keep teaching until spring vacation, but I might need to take a medical leave until next year, he thought I was jumping the gun and misinterpreting the facts. He wanted to wait and hear what the colorectal surgeon would have to say.

Thank goodness for the all the counselors in my life teaching me to take care of myself in situations like this. Through some flash of insight, I realized that we were both afraid, only reacting to the news in a different way. There is considerable strain on a relationship, in extreme times of stress, because of the conflicting ways that people need to deal with their fears. What I did was to return to my books and delve deeper for information. One thing was becoming clear to me: Our lives were going to be irrevocably changed by this latest news.

Stages of Colorectal Cancer

That afternoon, after research and reading, I learned that the size of a tumor was not as crucial to survival as much as how it behaved while it was in the body. To determine the seriousness of the disease, colorectal cancer is staged according to characteristics, involvement of lymph nodes, and metastases to other organs:

Stage One: The cancer has not gone beyond the inner lining of the bowel. Monitoring and removal of polyps is usually all that is needed for care. Survival statistics at this stage are in the 90% range.

Stage Two: The cancer has gone beyond the wall of the colon and traveled to a nearby tissue. In this case, surgical resection is necessary; radiation and chemotherapy may be recommended.

Stage Three: This is a more advanced stage where the cancer has invaded the lymph nodes. Resection, radiation, adjuvant chemotherapy are necessary. Survival statistics at this range are 30-70% for the first five years, if there is no recurrence.

Stage Four: If the cancer has come back close to an original site, it is called a "local recurrence." If it is at a distant site, such as the liver or the lung, it is called a "metastasis." Surgery at this level is largely to relieve symptoms and prolong life, although some cancers can still be cured if only a few metastases are present and surgery successfully removes all malignancy.

As I finished my reading, I put down my book and I stared out the window. With a setting sun, the water had grayness to it and those shimmering ripples had turned into more treacherous waves. I realized that I was in danger now and running for my life. I had plummeted downhill from Stage One to Stage Three in my journey with cancer.

**Tips for Travelers When the Diagnosis Changes

- Give yourself some time to adjust to your new diagnosis.
- Find the most positive person to talk to who will let you vent your feelings and help you form a new perspective.
- Become as well informed as you can about your type of cancer. Knowledge empowers you to make better decisions. The American Cancer Society and the National Institute of Health publish pamphlets that are loaded with information. Check Resources at the back of this book for addresses.
- Keep a journal. This can be a good source of therapy as you travel through each stage of your journey.
- Recognize people will accompany you on this part of the trip in different ways.

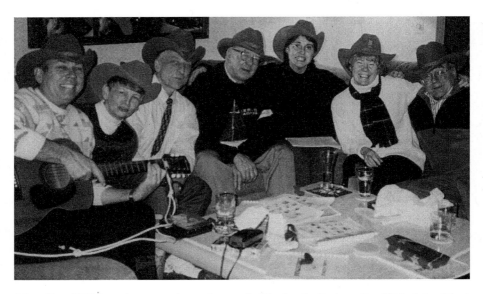

"Our Gang." We have been together so long we're like family. Rodney, Pat, Dick, John, Noni, me, and Dave celebrating Christmas. There is beauty and strength in the support of friends.

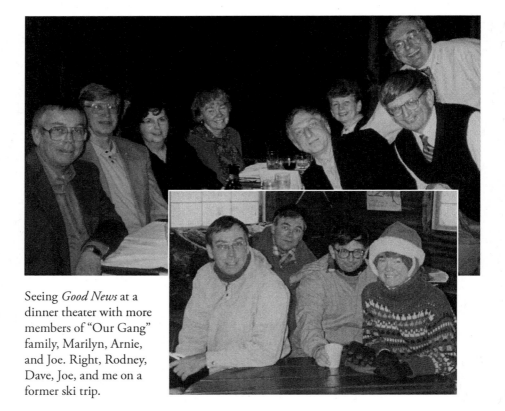

Seeing *Good News* at a dinner theater with more members of "Our Gang" family, Marilyn, Arnie, and Joe. Right, Rodney, Dave, Joe, and me on a former ski trip.

Chapter Four

Personal Concerns: Unexpected Problems

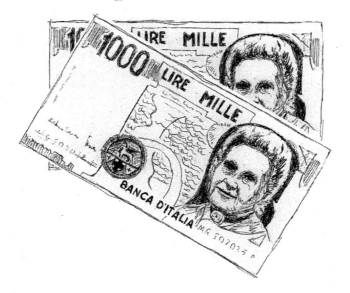

The bus is our home away from home. Huge, well ventilated and equipped with large windows, it is a comfortable way to travel. There are two seats on each side of the aisle, with room enough to turn around and talk to other people. The passengers are more familiar to us now. Our guide, Giulia, has a helpful way working with the group, which has fostered a feeling of camaraderie to the trip.

Our first stop-off is a gas and food super station along the road. With only 20 minutes reserved for this break, we visit the restrooms and try to order some refreshments. In haste, I join a line that moves too fast for me to figure out what I am going to order. I come up to the front, and quickly blurt out "uno cappuccino" trying to sound like one of the natives, but fooling no one. Instead of $2.00, I give the man $20.00 in Italian lire. It's only when I start to get back on the bus, I realize my mistake. Giulia is sympathetic, and goes back trying to retrieve the rest of my change, but returns with the message, "Is not possible."

I memorize the American equivalent to Italian money. This was a clear message of the importance of being informed. The stakes could be higher next time.

Later, that same day, during a rest break, Dave and I stop at an ATM machine. These are conveniently located all over Italy and are highly efficient in getting American dollars exchanged into new European money called "Euros." We put our cash card in, insert our PIN number, and discuss how much cash we want. Too late. Zap! The ATM machine sucks in our card like a vacuum and now it is irretrievable. Giulia, once again, regrettably tells us it "Is not possible" to get our card back, unless by mail. On top of that, the banks are closed for the day and closed tomorrow, which is Sunday.

If Dave and I were traveling alone, this potentially would be a real problem. As it is, our tour is taking care of our hotel room, breakfasts, and suppers. There are people on our bus, including Giulia, who offer to lend us money until Monday. Luckily, we are with friends who readily come up with the cash we need.

These were minor mishaps; however, this evening, after arriving at our hotel south of Pompeii in Sorrento, a young woman on our tour needs emergency medical care for a torn cornea. Giulia calls a doctor to get her pain medication and then arranges a driver to take the woman to Rome so she can see a specialist tomorrow.

There is beauty and strength in the support of other people when in a strange land or in trouble. This is true while you are visiting a foreign country, but it was also true for me when I was on my journey with cancer. People formed a caring network that helped every situation I encountered. Sometimes their concern came out in strange ways, but they meant well, anyway. This is the reason you will find cancer survivors, in particular, intent on dispersing random acts of kindness. We know how it feels to be isolated and alone, and the fortification that comes from the help of others.

Rerouting — Setting a New Course

Monday morning, after our trip to the North Shore, we had a consultation with the colorectal surgeon. I armed myself with knowledge and was determined to do anything necessary to regain my health.

First, I completed my first CT scan. This is a noninvasive diagnostic test to detect through X-rays if the disease had spread. In comparison to my other tests, the CT scan was a snap. It required drinking some radioactive dye and letting a machine detect if there were more traces of cancer. I was hoping the dye would behave itself and not go where I did not want it to go. I then carried the records with me as Dave, Red, and I met with the colorectal surgeon in his office.

The doctor was still just as direct and informative, but this time he was more resolute in impressing upon me the gravity of the situation.

"I want to make absolutely sure you know our plans have changed," he said emphatically. "We are now dealing with Stage Three of colorectal cancer."

Thankfully, I had already prepared myself emotionally for this fact before this conference. Dave, looking crestfallen, was now realizing what I had been trying to say to him up at the North Shore. The doctor continued, dispensing harsh information, educating us as we went along. After taking a painstakingly long look at my CT scan, he told me it came back negative.

"That's good," he said, "but I have to emphasize that this is an imprecise test."

He suggested, "You might want to go to another doctor for a second opinion."

While its wise to consider this possibility at this juncture of a diagnosis, I replied that I already felt I was working with a team of doctors and was confident I was going to get top-level care. As we talked more, I gathered up my nerve to ask him my most pressing question:

"What are my chances for survival?"

He looked at me square in the eye and said, "100%...because we're working with you and not a statistic."

Whether or not he has said this to numerous patients, it doesn't matter. What was significant was that he was saying it to me, sincerely, and it was powerful medicine for building my confidence. I would repeat this response over and over in the next two years, every time I would find myself on the edge of despair. I knew at that moment, this was the doctor I would choose to be my colorectal surgeon.

He then mapped out the current plan he was suggesting: five weeks of pre-operative radiation treatments, going every day, with three chemo treatments at the beginning, and three at the end; a resection taking out three-fourths of my rectum but leaving my colon, sphincter muscles, and bowel intact; further chemotherapy after I recovered from surgery.

Bypasses — Temporary Ostomies

So far, I had prepared myself for the doctor's prescriptive plan. Then there was the zinger. I would have to have a temporary ileostomy following surgery for at least six weeks.

"A what?" I asked.

"It's a bypass of your digestive system. A surgical opening created by a doctor in your abdominal wall. It will allow you to heal."

"Are you talking about a bag?" I had heard, through whispers, about those. At this point, my vanity took over. With all the other more hazardous kinds of treatment we had discussed, this by far bothered me the most. I wanted no more of this conversation, and started to consider that maybe, I would just hide my head in the sand and forget the whole thing.

He had obviously had this kind of resistance before, and he was ready for it. "It's probably going to be temporary, remember that," he repeated. "Most patients don't need a permanent ostomy. If everything goes according to plan, we will reverse the operation in six weeks."

"I tell you what I'm going to suggest. There are two enterostomal nurses at Fairview Hospital, Vicki and Julie, both excellent. They can give you more information. I think it will help if you go in and talk to either one of them."

In eight days I would start beginning treatments in chemotherapy and radiation. In about eight weeks I would be scheduled for surgery. All I could think about was the ileostomy and I was resistant. I didn't care how wonderful Vicki or Julie might be. I didn't want to see them, and I would not like anything they had to say. I went home with the attitude that this whole situation was becoming increasingly unfair. I had come a long way in accepting my new diagnosis and was prepared to start my treatments. I did not bargain for an ostomy.

First Aid — The Enterostomal Nurses

Despite my antagonistic feelings about the proposed ostomy, I made an appointment anyway with the enterostomal nurses. I knew that to refuse to have the resection would be too risky. I realized the importance of taking immediate action. Having a temporary ostomy was going to be part of this ordeal. I reluctantly decided to go in and at least get more information. I was scheduled to see Vicki the next day. When I arrived on the fourth floor of Fairview Hospital, both Vicki and Julie greeted me with unmistakable good will. Okay, I reasoned. They were likeable, but that didn't mean I had to like the fact that I was there. Vicki escorted me to one of the side rooms for a conference where we sat and talked. It felt as if I had a soothing companion at my side. She let me vent. She didn't try to deny that finding out I was going to have to have an ostomy was good news.

"I'm sorry. I've got a rotten attitude." I admitted. She came back with a voice that told me it was understandable for me to feel this way.

"Let me tell you what this is all about," Vicki suggested. I was ready to listen. Actually, I was curious.

She led me into the examining room filled with charts and supplies showing me quite a detailed chart on the colon and the upper, small intestine. It was one of the best maps of the human digestive system I have seen. By now, I was becoming somewhat of a connoisseur of digestive drawings. The small intestine is long – about 20 feet – and is coiled loosely in the abdomen.

After surgery, different types of ostomies are performed depending on how much and what part of the intestines is removed. In my case, the end of the lowest part of my small intestine, the ileum, would be brought out of my abdominal wall. This is called a "stoma" and it is reddish pink in color. There is no valve to shut this off. Digestive material would pass through my body and into my stoma on a continuous basis into a pouch, which I would always have to wear as long as I had the ileostomy. I grimaced.

Vicki picked up on my reaction, and kept reassuring me to stay with her, as she explained the rest. She then showed me the first picture I had ever seen of a stoma. It was so small and so unprotected, it hardly could take the role of the ugly monster I had in mind. The bags she showed me, which I had denounced in the colorectal surgeon's office, were more the size of a small sandwich variety. They were white, disposable, would be attached by an adhesive to my skin, and would be completely sanitary. But what of the reality? Would there be an odor when I was out in public? What kind of clothes would I have to wear?

She assured me that when I was with other people, no one would have to be aware I was even wearing an appliance. Spandex, body-clinging shorts, maybe, would be out for me. I replied that at my age, they were out for me, anyway. The idea that no one would ever have to know appealed to me. I could keep my secret buried forever. These new disposable bags were efficient and would keep me odor-free. Emptying them regularly with water would prevent telltale bulges.

I got the clear message that having an ostomy would be just as bad or as good as I made it. The adjustment was up to the individual. While she was not minimizing my concerns, she was certainly helping to take the sting out of them. Julie came in again to see how everything was going, and the three of us engaged in a conversation about my colorectal surgeon and the practice of which he was a member. Their positive comments reaffirmed my feelings of confidence, plus they readily endorsed the oncologist and radiation specialist that were recommended to me.

I left their office with hope. I was surprised at what a turnaround my attitude had taken. Now I was feeling "lucky." Not to have cancer, certainly. Not to have to have an ileostomy. But if I was going to have to take such a journey, I felt like I had been placed on this superhighway of caregivers. I would not be abandoned on a lonely road. People who I felt were trustworthy were taking my hand, leading the way to a safer place.

Well-wishers — Saying, "Bon Voyage"

While I was waiting to begin my treatments, I coped with my negative feelings with bravado as much as I could. My mother used to be like that. Ten years ago, when she was alive and in her 90's, I remember standing in line at the grocery store watching her as she told the checkout girl she was going to be moving to a new assisted-living apartment. She covered up her fears by making it sound like she was ready for whatever life had in store for her. I was trying to do the same thing by telling others that I was bravely facing up to what I was going to have to go through.

Late at night, however, if I happened to wake up, I couldn't shake off my anxieties. I worried about the fact I was about ready to voluntarily poison myself with chemicals, jeopardize my immune system, and destroy some of the healthy cells in my body. I would pull the blankets over my head and bury myself in my pillow for comfort. I knew at those moments I was plenty scared and I was already grieving for the healthy body that had been left behind. Still, during the day, talking to other people buoyed my confidence and made me feel less alone in this experience.

This path of being open with people worked well for me most of the time. I soon discovered how many lives of the people I knew had been touched by cancer. Other people sought me out for information, particularly about what a colonoscopy was like and how did I discover I was sick in the first place? While I felt that I was doing some good by talking to them, I soon learned that others did not want to talk about any kind of cancer, especially colorectal cancer. For those people, I tried to stay away from bringing up the subject of my health. Not even David Letterman could get many people to include rectal matters on their favorite top ten lists of conversational topics.

One head-on collision I found unavoidable. I was standing in the hall of our school, having a conversation with one of the teachers in our building, responding to her questions about my situation, when one of the coaches walked by. He stopped and listened in to what I was saying.

"What's wrong with you?" he butted in.

I flinched.

"I…have colorectal cancer."

He laughed. Not really a laugh of glee, but discomfort. His discomfort. Then he shook his head with annoyance and walked on, not saying another word. Obviously, I had been too blunt.

The teacher I had been talking to was appalled. She was a sympathetic sort and wanted to let me know she was offended.

"That was terrible for him to act that way."

"Well, I probably caught him off-guard."

"Oh, but, Carol, that was awful," she continued, "I mean, you're going to die aren't you?"

Now I had to laugh and I was the one feeling discomfort.

"Gee, I hope not," I managed to say. "At least, that's not my intention. The odds are pretty much in my favor not to have that happen."

She nodded and said, "Oh, good."

The tone of her voice said, however, that she was not convinced. I had to leave. I walked out of the building immediately and hurried home to look upon my garden.

Ways That People Can Help

Why couldn't everyone say or do the right thing? If Giulia had been there, she would've said, "Is not possible."

My family kept me grounded and provided a safety net for me in different ways. Tami, my oldest daughter, found all the information that she could and set up a schedule for cleaning if I needed to have things done at home. Laura, the middle child, kept me distracted with her wedding plans. She was also completing her Master's Degree and asked me to be her "Capstone Advisor" so I was reading and editing her research. My husband, Dave, trying to create a world of normalcy when I talked to him, was hoping to convince me (and himself) that nothing much would change. My youngest daughter, Jenny, became like a trainer, encouraging me to build up my strength. My cousin, Meg, a therapist in Marin County, California, became my personal guidance counselor. Meg's mother, my aunt Jean, my brother Red, and his wife, Sandy, kept me company while I was preparing myself for what was to come.

All of these approaches were helpful, although at times I know I resisted some of their efforts. It felt uncomfortable for me to accept that I might need the help of my children. Sometimes Meg and I differed about the way we viewed alternative methods of healing. I did not always want a guidance counselor…or a teacher…or a trainer. Sometimes I wished that Dave and I could talk more about the potential dangers that were ahead.

Other people reacted in different ways to my predicament, but relayed messages of hope and caring concern. I went into my dentist's office to get a good cleaning and they suggested a fluoride treatment and nonalcoholic mouthwash to prevent me from getting mouth sores from the chemo. Afterward, I received an exquisite orchid from Noni, my friend and hygienist, who said it would keep blooming until after surgery. Later, that week, the whole dental staff sent me flowers with a wish for good luck.

There was a long list of dear friends who came forward with their prayers, their inspiration, and gifts from the heart: baked goodies, flowers, a delicately painted pillow for me to place over me when I slept, a dream catcher, specially written letters, or email messages, and others who let me know in different ways they "were there for me" by just listening to my concerns as we sat in restaurants, or gathered in each other's homes.

Our Gang, my second family, took Dave and me to a dinner theater, where they were presenting the play, "Good News." It was the night before I went in for my first treatments, and they correctly guessed that the music and the upbeat nature of the play would be good medicine. After the play, we had a "group hug" and then there they stood, waving goodbye to me, as if I were going on a very long trip, which of course, was true. I might be facing a hazardous journey, but the send-offs I was getting from all these people cushioned my anxieties.

**Tips for Travelers When You Need Support

- Keep your sense of humor. It will restore your humanity.
- Accept the help of your friends and family. Recognize that people will accompany you on this part of the trip in different ways.
- Seek help. Find a good therapist or someone who cares about you who will allow you to vent your feelings while helping you to get to a better place.
- Most hospitals will offer support groups dealing with all aspects of cancer. There are also some excellent sources of help that can be accessed by going online such as colon@listserv.acor.org and www.cancer.org
- The magazines, *Coping With Cancer* P.O. Box 682268, Franklin, TN 37068-2268, and *Cure* 3535 Worth Street, Dallas TX 75246 have inspirational articles and information about all different types of cancer. *Stressfree Living* offers articles on health and lifestyle topics, 14070 Commerce Ave. Suite 200, Prior Lake, MN 55372 or go to www.stressfreeliving.org.
- If you are in need of information about an ostomy, call UOAA at 1-800-826-0826, the United Ostomy Associations of America, Inc. They will send you information and help you find a support group in your area. Their website is www.uoaa.org.
- The OAMA, Ostomy Association of the Minneapolis Area, offers education, a nonprofit support program, and a newsletter. P.O. Box 385453, Bloomington, MN 55438-5453.
- The UOAA publishes a quarterly magazine *The Phoenix,* P.O. Box 3605, Mission Vejo, CA 92690 www.uoaa.org.
- Check the last chapter in this book about support groups, www.getyourrearingear.com and C3, info@fightcolorectal.org.

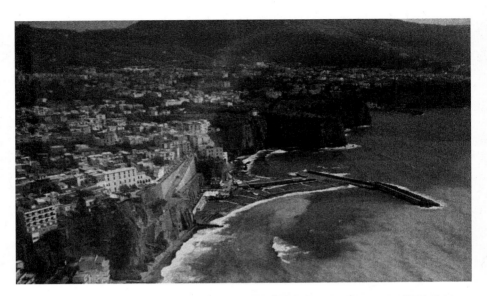

The Amalfi Coast
gave us pictures
worth remembering.

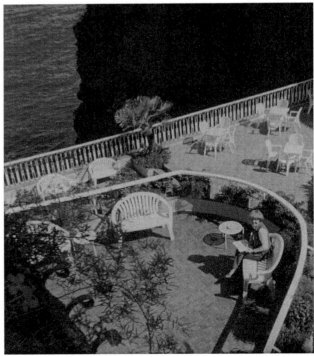

CHAPTER FIVE

The Value of a Beautiful Outlook: The Amalfi Coast

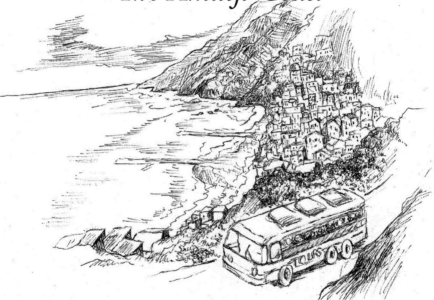

Traveling south of Pompeii, we approach the Amalfi Coast. This is a 48-mile stretch along the Italian Mediterranean Sea from Sorrento to Salerno, described in our tour book as one of the most beautiful drives in the world. While that statement may be true, it also is surely one of the most dangerous. With a 500-foot drop to the water, it feels like we are flying rather than traveling on a bus. Cars are racing by on a narrow two-lane highway at such a speed we expect them to take off in the air. We trust that our bus driver knows what he is doing. Like small children, we press our faces to the windows and look out in wonder.

I am grateful for what I know about photography, as I am framing pictures with my eyes. The afternoon light is reflected on small toy-like villages nestled in the limestone cliffs along the way. The turquoise watercolors of the Mediterranean, the contrasting lemon and olive trees, and the sandy coves below all blend together in harmony like a well composed picture. I have learned to memorize each scene of beauty in my mind and store it as a picture in an album. Then, on days when there is no sunshine, no colorful landscape, I can recapture the pleasure of any panorama. Some of these beautiful pictures I think of now are of the people who have helped me survive my journey with cancer, making me feel less fearful along the way. With a little imagination, almost any experience becomes easier to endure through the use of imagery.

The First Introduction to Chemotherapy

Just like approaching the edge of a 500-foot drop, heading toward chemo and radiation treatments dominated my outlook on life. There were fleeting moments when I felt I was about ready to plunge over a cliff into an abyss of nameless agonies, from which I would emerge at the very least, psychologically damaged and spent. There were times I found it hard to sit back and merely act the part of a passenger, taken care of by more expert drivers.

Part of the problem before people begin chemotherapy and radiation treatments is that there are very few positive pictures of what this experience is like to help them get through that first initial encounter. As I opened the door to the oncologist's office for chemotherapy, I felt like I might be walking into a den of torment where victims would be submissively waiting for their turn in the chamber of horrors. This was hardly the case. The waiting room looked like any other doctor's office. Most of the patients were reading magazines or talking with each other in pleasant conversations. The only difference I could see was that there was coffee, cookies, and hard candies available.

When I met the oncologist, he hardly seemed to fit the role of a persecutor. For one thing, he was casually dressed in Dockers and a trendy deep blue denim shirt. He had a disarming, easygoing way about him that seemed like he was miscast for this part that I had assigned him to play. We discussed my records, and the progression of my illness seriously enough, but when he asked me if I had any questions and saw my list, there was a slight grin on his face.

"You typed your list?" he asked.

On cue, I dutifully replied, "I'm a special education teacher and we learn to keep good records."

He nodded with reserved amusement. "I've just never had a patient do that before," he explained. "Okay… so, what did you want to know?"

"What will be my schedule of treatments?" My heart was beating a little faster on this one.

"Before your operation, starting today, we will give you three treatments on Monday, Tuesday and Wednesday followed by three more daily doses at the end of radiation. After surgery, you'll be given a dose of chemotherapy once a week, in six week cycles, with two weeks off for a vacation."

I slumped my shoulders and let out a sigh.

"What are the side effects?"

"It's not going to be all that bad," he assured me. He explained that these drugs were not going to be as devastating as other forms of chemotherapy. I was told I probably would not lose my hair, but might get some mouth sores. The nausea would more than likely be mild and they had drugs to counteract it. I would be tired, but I could continue to work if I wanted to.

I was pleasantly surprised by this news and beginning to lose a grip on my fears, the more he talked. We discussed my treatment, a combination of something called leucovorin and 5FU.

"What do you call it?" I was sure I hadn't heard him correctly.

"5FU. Stands for fluorouracil. That's what we suggest along with the leucovorin."

I have a weird sense of humor that springs up at odd moments, much to my embarrassment. I tried not to laugh, but I did anyway.

"Sorry," I said. "I've been a high school teacher too long. FU has another meaning for me."

The chemo doctor picked up on what I was referring to and grinned wryly, "High school's a different world, isn't it? But here, FU stands for fluorouracil."

I went back to my list. "How long will each treatment be? From what I have heard it takes between 4-6 hours."

"That's what it used to be. Now it will take about 5 minutes to inject it into your veins, with about 10 minutes of intravenous solution to water it down." When he saw my obvious relief at this news, he teased, "They made it better just for you."

By the time our conference was over, I had lost much of my dread. We proceeded to the room where I was to get my treatments. There were about nine patients sitting in olive green leather chaise lounges circling the nurse's station, hooked up to intravenous machines. Most of the people appeared healthy, even though a few faces seemed set as if they were stoically enduring some sort of hardship. Some people were sleeping and others were talking. I noticed one person in the corner who looked jaundiced and had a fragile, sickly body with a worn expression on his face. Right there in that room, I found all the evidence I needed that there was a difference in severity of chemotherapy treatments.

The nurses on duty greeted me warmly. They must have been hand picked for being upbeat and empathetic and that helped. I sat down in one of the lounge chairs, and we talked pleasantly, as they explained the procedures, while my hand was quickly turned into a pincushion, trying to find the best vein.

After the initial thrust of intravenous fluids, I felt a mildly hot sensation as the poison was administered into my system. A metallic taste in my mouth accompanied the invasion. Within 20 minutes, I was done. That was it. The first dose was anticlimactic. I did not feel any particular effect at all except for a mild awareness that I had something foreign injected into my bloodstream that my body didn't like. That reaction probably was part emotion, and part physical. I walked out of there feeling fairly normal and made my way over to the hospital where I would get my first dosage of radiation.

Radiation

I heard from other people that "radiation wasn't bad" so I wasn't as fearful about this part of my treatment. The radiation doctor was a distinguished looking gentleman with white hair and glasses who had a reassuring way about him.

He explained that high-energy radiation I would be exposed to for the next six weeks would not be painful, except for side effects that might develop. Because of the area treated, diarrhea and some loss of appetite were to be expected. He assured me that with medication, these symptoms could be minimized. Skin irritation might be a problem, especially with the fact that I was a redhead and had always been sensitive to the sun. Fatigue might be experienced during the last three weeks. These symptoms would more than likely disappear as soon as my treatments were over.

Some people did develop more chronic side effects, he explained, but he didn't think that I would be one of them. I bought into that argument. I reasoned if chemotherapy would not be that bad, radiation probably wouldn't give me much trouble. Any other warnings I got from the literature they handed out were so generalized that it was like the soft voice-over accompanying the TV ad in the background of an upbeat picture. If you ever took what was being said seriously, realizing it might apply to you, you'd never in your right mind buy into the product.

After our conference, when I walked into the radiation room, my first thought was "You've got to be kidding." The only thing I could compare it to was a movie set of a 50's sci-fi drama where the heroine was about to be transported to some distant planet. The room was darkened. Before me was a gigantic white plastic beamer approximately 20 feet high.

I removed all clothes from the waist down, was told to climb a footstool, and to lie face down under an X-ray machine. As a test run, the exact area where I was to be radiated was pinpointed and marked. I was given a painless temporary tattoo with semi-permanent ink that I was told could withstand bathing, but not rubbing, and would remain on my left buttock for the rest of the six weeks.

The procedure required that they leave me alone in the room for my treatments because it would be too damaging to them to stay in the room. That should have told me something. They did assure me that they would be monitoring the whole process and that it would last just a few minutes.

I was lying face down, but I could hear the whirring of the machine as it radiated me and beamed down on the chosen spot in my anal area. I was told to breathe normally and not move. I tried not to imagine I was going to be transported to Mars. As opposed to that scenario, I started to fantasize I was in a microwave oven being nuked with rays. That thought terrified me, so I switched to imagining I was just in a tanning booth getting bronzed, and that image worked for me.

Before I knew it, it was over, and I was given a special parking stamp allowing me to pull right up to the curb in front of the radiation door. I went home pleased with the way that I had faced up to all I was encountering that first day, relieved that it was over.

I finished two other days of chemo with just a mild feeling of nausea, and proceeded in the next two weeks to drive myself to the hospital for radiation treatments every day after work, hop on the table, receive my "tanning session" and return home. As it was, for the first two weeks, I was wondering what all the fuss was about. I didn't have much of a reaction to the chemotherapy treatments and I wasn't getting any reaction from the radiation. In fact, I was joking about my "tanning" booth.

My life formed a predictable pattern. Every day, at 3:00 p.m. when I finished teaching school, I would drive over to the hospital, park in a spot reserved for radiation patients, go in and get "zapped." I became very agile at doing this, and the nurses kidded me I was setting records for getting on and off the table so quickly. While I was getting my treatments I would imagine a beautiful scene, such as the water lapping up on the rocks of the North Shore, and think of myself lying there enjoying the sunshine.

This was a time of self indulgence and euphoria for me. I ate whatever I felt like eating. Now that I was done with the first dosages of chemo and actually receiving radiation, it was so painless I felt rather free of fear. People went out of their way to be kind to me and I was particularly kind to myself. I drove to my radiation treatments after school and played Lord of the Dance and Andrea Bocelli's *Romanza*. The sunrises that greeted me each morning seemed especially iridescent with their pearl-like charm. I continued to wear my Irish Claddaugh ring for luck.

Two weeks rushed by, and finally we were breaking for our school's spring vacation. I had already put in for sick leave, so I knew I was not coming back for the rest of the year. The day had been nice but uneventful. I looked around at my empty room, and I had a flashing, frightening thought. What if I never would be coming back? Just then, my principal came into the room and we reminisced over all the memories of teaching we both shared through the years. Dave showed up to pick up my boxes and Laura, my coworker, suggested we go out for a drink. That was it. I closed the door behind me on the classroom I had loved and walked out of the school.

By the third week, I was still not having many side effects. I was even questioning my decision about not returning to work after vacation was over. The only trouble I was having was not being hungry and losing my appetite. Gradually, without realizing it, I was also cutting down on fluids. Not a good thing to do! I was experiencing some gastric upsets and taking almost daily medication for diarrhea. Every day, to lessen the effects of radiation, I was supposed to take sitz baths at home. Still trying to infuse some pleasure into this situation, I imagined I was at a spa, filled the bathroom with candles, and soaked in the bathtub.

By the fourth week, however, the scene changed. I was nauseated quite often and extremely tired. I did not know at the time about the devastating effects dehydration could have on the body and wasn't aware this condition was probably giving me additional problems. All of my lower organs had become tender. My bodily functions and bouts of diarrhea were causing me some discomfort, but I also was becoming listless and feeling vulnerable. I was determined to complete all my treatments, regardless. I went in for my final pre-surgery chemo booster shots, which probably lowered my resistance.

When I went in the last week, the nurses kept asking me if I would be able to withstand further radiation, as they could see the area being treated was becoming quite blistered and red. I felt like I was in that microwave oven again, being over-cooked. I knew that was a negative image, but the tanning booth analogy didn't work anymore.

The last day of my radiation treatment I was disappointed to find out my regular doctor was off for the week and I was assigned another radiation doctor. This one was an attractive female, young enough to be my daughter, who I initially related to quite well. As two women talking to each other, I found it easy to be explicit about the irritability and soreness I was feeling in my bladder and while urinating.

"Is this a burning sensation?" she asked.

"No." I replied, "but in the past this is way I felt at the beginning of a yeast infection or a bladder infection, so I was thinking that's what's happening to me now."

"You'd be having more of an acute pain if that was the case" she determined. Too quickly, I thought. "The symptoms you're having are due to the culmination of your radiation treatments."

She was the doctor, her voice said, and I was the patient. I shouldn't be doing the diagnosing. Case closed.

"Isn't this dangerous, giving people this heavy of a dosage?" I persisted.

The doctor measured her words as she replied, "Well, we want to insure the radiation is doing its work. Probably all symptoms will vanish with time. Of course, there may be lasting side effects."

"Such as?" I asked with a feeling of dread.

"Oh, some people may have permanent damage to the rectum. In that case, you'd have chronic pain, but I wouldn't worry about it."

I blinked. I couldn't believe what I was hearing and the way this information was being communicated to me. It seemed so nonchalant. I could not help but wonder if permanent damage to my rectum would interfere with my ileostomy reversal. I wanted to ask her about this outcome, but I was too upset. I knew better than to kill the messenger, but I felt she could have delivered her information with more sensitivity. My mind tried to deal with the fact that this might be an outcome. Again, not for everyone. Possibly me.

I tried to stifle my reactions. I could worry about this later, but I was obviously not happy with this news. I was feeling so sick at this point, I wasn't very happy anyway. I went back to the discomfort that I was feeling at the moment and once again asked her if I should be in so much pain.

By this time, she appeared to be irritated and done with conference.

"It would be easy enough to just give you a test to find out if you have another infection, but it probably would be a waste of time."

She closed her files on me and prepared to stand as a signal that my time was up. "I won't order any other tests unless you insist on them."

I was wishing I could talk to my regular doctor. I was feeling weak, but I was overwhelmed. I hung my head and said with resignation, "No, that's not necessary." I left the room, went in for my final radiation treatment, trying not to burst into tears, and went home.

I felt miserable and achy the whole next day. I tried to tell myself I would feel better with time, but instead I became progressively worse. Later the following night, I experienced sharp, burning sensations as I passed my urine. I went into the emergency room and was diagnosed with a whopping yeast infection. I was given strong medication for the problem and went to bed for the next couple of days. We left for my daughter's cabin in Aitkin, Minnesota that weekend, so I could get some rest. By Sunday, however, I was not getting much better.

I was dismayed that the medication I was taking wasn't doing its job. Once again, I went in to another emergency room, this time in Aitkin.

A quick test revealed a rather advanced urinary infection, which luckily had not traveled any further to my kidneys. Had I just taken medication a few days earlier, however, I could have avoided all the pain that was now searing through my whole system.

It would take me a week to finally feel better. As soon as the diarrhea stopped and my infections cleared up, my resiliency slowly returned. I would have to contend with some adverse effects of radiation damage to my rectum later.

My ability to conjure up a beautiful picture, giving me a respite from all the turmoil I felt inside, was a skill that served me well while I was recuperating, just as it had during radiation.

Looking back, I know I should have trusted my instincts. I should have persisted in my complaints and insisted on having additional tests. I could have postponed my last radiation treatments until I could talk to my regular radiation doctor and perhaps lessened dire side effects that would affect me later. This was my first real lesson in learning that I had to listen to what my body was saying above all else. I would be learning that lesson over and over again in the next year.

Myths About Radiation

There are some myths people have about radiation. One of the most prevalent is that a person becomes radioactive. What actually happens is that energy is converted into a biochemical change, while radiation injures or destroys the DNA of selective cells. All people do not react the same to radiation, just as all people do not react the same to the sun's rays. The other myth that exists is that radiation is harmless. While the risks of side effects are less than the benefit of killing the cancer cells, keep in mind that radiation is a powerful treatment. Ask about all the possible side effects of the treatments that might affect you as an individual, and realize that you can put a stop to them when you feel that you have had enough.

**Tips for Travelers During Radiation and Chemotherapy:

• Research side effects of each cancer treatment before you see the doctor.
• Ask questions. You have the right to be informed.
• Dehydration can become a problem. Take seriously the suggestion that you should drink at least 8 glasses of water a day.
• Make sure you are getting enough nutrition in your diet. Supplemental vitamins may be helpful on this trek of the journey.
• Consult your dentist about preventative measures. A fluoride treatment and non-alcoholic mouthwash may help prevent mouth sores.
• Take sitz baths. They are both relaxing and therapeutic.
• If you are experiencing pain, or worried about possible outcomes of your treatment, consult a doctor who will listen to you.

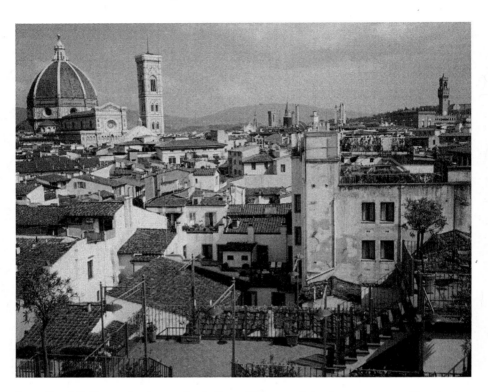

Brunelleschi's Dome dominates the skyline of Florence. It has been a source of inspiration since the Middle Ages.

CHAPTER SIX

The Power of Inspiration: The Duomo

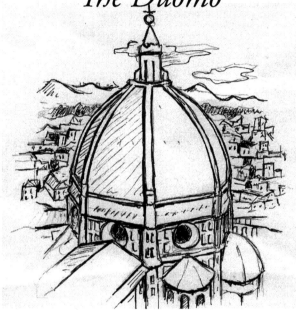

We travel inland going north through the Italian countryside to Florence. From our hotel we can look at the sunset superimposing a brilliant glow to Florence's most prominent cathedral, nicknamed "The Duomo." From a height of 366 feet, looking like a burnt orange terra cotta bishop's hat, the dome of the church dominates the skyline. The next day, we take a short walk to Cathedral Square, religious center of Florentine life since the Middle Ages where the Italian Renaissance began. Entering the huge cathedral of the Duomo, the gray harshness of medieval architecture surrounds us until we step into the sanctuary, and walk under Brunelleschi's dome. We look up at a huge cupola that vaults to heights of glory. For a brief moment, we are lifted into another magnificent world, far beyond the realities of this one. I can imagine the awe felt by the populace coming to this church inspired by this wonder.

Amazing how one person can inspire so many others. At the beginning of the Renaissance, in 1418, Brunelleschi had previously established a reputation for himself by applying the principles of perspective to painting. He then proceeded to do the same thing with his original design for the Duomo as a way to vault space. He faced fierce competition and derision for his plan, but it turned out to be a masterpiece and changed the history of architecture forever. The height and span of his dome was unsurpassed until the 20th century and only then by using modern materials.

The Duomo was meant to inspire and restore faith, but you don't have to go to Italy for that purpose. After my surgery was over, I found out that inspiration could be found from many sources and reach you anywhere, even in a hospital room. Struggling with my worse moments, I came to realize that my spiritual understanding of the idea of "something beyond" our human existence was simply the endurance of love. It was a revelation that was to give my recovery amazing grace. I would also discover the inspirational role caregivers would take on in determining how I would view my present situation.

Surgery

I was scheduled for surgery the third week in May. I was less afraid of this part of my journey because of my past experiences of childbirth and other operations. I learned, with proper medication, the actual surgery and recovery time in the hospital probably would be manageable for me.

Finally, the day arrived when I checked into the hospital and was prepped for my operation. I was then rolled down the hallway on a cart. My children and Dave were by my side, making small talk and joking with me. When the door of the elevator opened, and we tearfully said our "good-byes", it was as if all the years we had been together were being placed on an altar, as an offering of our lives.

Would life ever be the same again? Just for a brief moment, I wanted to get off of the cart and become a spectator to this scene, rather than a participant in the service. Then I was wheeled into the elevator and was lifted up to another floor accompanied by an orderly pushing me into a new existence.

Seeing an operating room from the perspective of the operating table, I looked up onto acoustic white ceiling panels and glaring lights. I was surrounded by walls that had pale ceramic tiles reminding me more of a huge bathroom than a place where an operation was going to take place. People in the room, of course, were at an angle to my vision, which gave them a heightened appearance, like they were floating in space. They were preparing themselves to delve into my body, and just for a moment, I was not sure I was going to give them permission to do that. Then I heard the commanding voice of my colorectal surgeon. As he looked down to greet me, he asked, "Are you ready?"

I nodded. I knew at that minute I was going to cooperate, as much as I could. Actually, the word, "cooperate" is a wonderfully descriptive word for this moment. I became part of the operating team and said a silent prayer as the anesthesiologist put me to sleep. I thought to myself, this has to be the epitome of trust…and then all was oblivion.

Sanctuary After Surgery

For the next 24 hours, I can't remember being in pain. I must have been, of course, considering that six inches of my rectum was removed, but I can't remember it. I was well attended to and kept warm. I even was coaxed into getting up and walking the next day.

I was given the choice of a private room as I was expected to be in the hospital for at least five more days. It upped the cost of my stay slightly, but the expense was well worth it. Gradually, I was weaned off morphine by using a patient-controlled device that administered medication only when I needed it. As my state of awareness increased, I was able to talk to my family again, almost as if I had never left their side.

There were telltale signs I had been on an eventful trip, however. I had a significant incision across my abdomen, and a new stoma, enclosed in a transparent plastic bag. It wasn't functioning just yet, but I knew it was there and would have to remain there for at least six weeks. I was told the operation was a success, but it would take a few days to find out if any other malignancies had been discovered. I slept quite a bit of the time.

By the second day I recovered enough to have visitors. I was off of the heavy stuff, but still taking powerful pain pills. People were calling me on the phone and stopping in to see me. I was having lots of good, short conversations with the staff.

All this attention was gratifying, but overwhelming, too. I found it exhausting to be so "sociable." Every time I went into the bathroom, I had to face the scars of my surgery and the new appliance hanging from my belly. It was no worse than having a Ziplock bag taped onto your stomach, but it bothered me, nevertheless. That night I hardly slept. I was taut like a rubber band and especially talkative when the nurses came in to check me.

By morning I was exhausted and over-stimulated. My colorectal surgeon made his rounds and was not pleased when he heard how I was doing.

"Sleep is restorative, you know," he admonished.

"I've tried, but I can't seem to settle down. The nurses come in and I start talking to them. The phone keeps on ringing, and I suppose I've been having too much company."

"We can fix that," he said decisively. Shazzam. Captain Marvel had my phone disconnected. I was given a mild sleeping pill, and when I woke up there was a sign on my door declaring, "Absolutely NO visitors — including staff!"

The "me" who has always loved company breathed easier. Not having to put up a brave front was a relief. Being alone with myself was just what I needed. I got to cry. I had the luxury of being in a funk. I didn't even put on any make-up, which was unusual for me. I retreated from the world. I felt protected.

Inspirational Visitors

The following day, I wondered if God had summoned some additional help. Even allowing for the fact that I had been on heavy painkillers, and that I was very needy, I had an experience that exceeded any rational explanation I could invent. I was completely lucid, and knew exactly where I was, and to whom I was talking.

In the back of my bed were some outlets and electrical devices. However, what I saw reflected in my blank television screen was reconfigured by me to be my mother as a young nurse monitoring my vital signs. I could look in the back of me, and see what was really there. It didn't matter.

When I looked up, my mother was diligently keeping watch over me. To the right of me, were some flowers. In the TV screen, they formed a picture of my Uncle Bob and my Aunt Ethel in their old age. All of these people had been dead for years. My mom died at 92, Ethel at 98, and Bob died at 88. They had been very good friends in real life and were having a wonderful time being together now, visiting, laughing and joking.

I was at the center of this group, but in reality I was in my bed looking upon myself. I tried to import other people like my Aunt Jean and my brother, but I could only imagine they were there for short intervals and then they disappeared. I saw myself lying there, in my robe and wearing sunglasses.

As strange as this sounds, I believe I needed sunglasses because the light was so bright. It was dazzling. This all seemed perfectly natural to me. I wasn't afraid or even thinking this was crazy. What was conveyed, along with their images, was a loving, soothing aura. Nothing bad was going to hurt me. Not right now. I was safe.

My daughter and my granddaughter came to see me that same evening around supper. (They were allowing me to have visitors from my family now, by my request.) They were there for a few minutes, and then, Tami asked, "Mom, what are you looking at?" She noticed that I kept looking at the blank screen of my TV set. It was turned off. I felt a little strange telling her what I was seeing. I could hardly understand it myself.

After I told Tami what I was seeing, she looked steadily at me, and said, "I'll call you when I get home." That night, this is what she related. My granddaughter, Courtney, was almost four at the time, and a very sensitive child.

When she and Tami had entered my hospital room, Courtney whispered, "Who are all these people in here? It's so crowded."

Tami was perplexed. There was no one else in the room that she could see. "Courtney," she said, "What do you mean? There's no one else here but Grandma."

Courtney then corrected her. "Oh yes. There's lots of people. Some of them are dead and some are alive."

I have heard of these things happening to other people, never taking them too seriously, but after this experience have been less skeptical. I believe I was given a spiritual glimpse of something wonderful beyond any human explanation. I have kept these images in my memory ever since, and they bring me into a peaceful, loving state. It has altered significantly my concept of love transcending life. What a gift.

The next day, the images vanished, and I felt much stronger. The TV screen was blank. No matter how much I wanted to bring back the previous images, I couldn't do it, except from memory. I was able to cut way down on medication.

By late afternoon of the fourth day, I felt better. I ate some real food, and was digesting it properly. Both Vicki and Julie, my enterostomal therapists, had been my exclusive visitors taking turns coming in to see me. We had already established good rapport, so I could tell them about my reactions and how I was adjusting to my new ileostomy. They were fascinated by my story of my deceased relatives "visiting me" the day before. Those images lessened my fears, but I was still struggling with my feelings about the ostomy.

"What's wrong with me anyway?" I asked Vicki tearfully.

"Carol, you've been through a lot, and your body has been altered. You need to give yourself permission to grieve. Makes perfect sense to me."

I needed a hug and she gave it to me. Later, Julie came in and also gave me some more positive reinforcement. Talking to both of them, I tried to joke about it, making references to my "carryout" bag and needing no more emergency runs into the bathroom. How glad I was that it was just temporary. How strange it was that I didn't want to see or talk to anybody.

They gave me some tips on rinsing my pouch with water, and brought me deodorizing drops that would take care of unwanted aromas while changing my pouch.

We talked and made jokes about other factors of hospital life. With my permission, they were going to arrange for someone from the Ostomy Foundation to come in and talk to me. It was like being sprinkled with faerie dust. Enterostomal therapists do so much more than just give out medical advice.

They are in a strategic position to guide patients when they are feeling incredibly lost.

After lunch, a beautiful young woman walked into my room and introduced herself. I was wondering who she was, and why was she there. Then she explained that she had an ostomy. She was requested by Vicki and Julie to come and see me. She sat down and we swapped stories about all the difficulties we both have had adjusting to a new apparatus.

We talked about how hard it is to have your body image change and live with it that way. Five years ago, after a severe colitis attack, she had to have an emergency operation just before her wedding. My heart went out to her. It was one thing to contend with this at my age, but at 24? It was therapeutic for me to see how well she was doing now. It was at this point that I made a mental note to work on my attitude. This one person helped me to take three giant steps in overcoming the depressing feelings I had adjusting to my ostomy. Someday, I vowed, I would do the same for someone else.

I had two other significant visitors before I went home. One night after supper, the gastroenterologist, the man who had performed my initial colonoscopy stopped in to see me and check up on how I was doing. He glanced around my room and then looked out the window. He seemed to want to say more to me, so I just sat back and waited.

"This room," he said with emotion, "Is the same room I was in. For surgery."

"Really?" I replied. "That must feel eerie to you."

He sighed. "It sure does. I was diagnosed with cancer ten years ago. And here I am."

I was extremely touched that he should take the time to tell me this and I told him so. He gave me hope that I, too, could recover.

"I just wanted you to know that people do survive cancer and go on to productive lives," he said and then left the room.

My colorectal surgeon came to check me out the last day I was in the hospital, and to give me the biopsy results from my operation. I was conscious during this time that my prognosis was "on hold" until I knew what the score would be. When he started to read me his findings, I was aware that my heart was racing and my nerves were on edge.

"Everything proceeded as we predicted." He paused after this statement and said, "but of course, there is evidence of metastatic adenocarcinoma spreading to the lymph nodes."

I didn't move. I felt my whole body tighten up. "S…s…so, what happens now?"

When he saw the look on my face, and heard the quiver in my voice, he added, "But these are the nodes we saw in your original ultrasound. It doesn't appear there are any more."

I was choked up; all I could murmur was an unintelligible, "Oh."

"It looks like at this point, you are cancer free."

"Cancer free." Those words changed my perspective immediately. My spirits soared. I broke into tears but I was smiling at the news and feeling overjoyed.

"We're still suggesting that you go back to the oncologist and complete the other chemotherapy. We can talk later whether you want to do this before or after your reversal."

At that moment, I felt like I had been given dispensation from the Pope, being told that I could now leave and go home. A surge of relief, like a spiritual baptism, was washing over me.

I stumbled over words trying to explain how grateful I was for everything he accomplished. I didn't have to say that much however, because I am sure he knew.

He then proceeded to give me instructions. He would send home some pain pills. I needed to rest, and be on a low residue diet. We made another appointment and then he pleasantly left me to absorb all the information I had heard. I was going home. I wouldn't be getting any more treatments until after Laura's wedding, seven weeks from my discharge from the hospital. He left the room. I said a prayer to my mom, Ethel, and Bob thanking them for watching over me. I felt they were celebrating too.

Tips For Travelers Having Surgery:

- Read and follow all directions while preparing for surgery.
- Optimism, the power of prayer, and a willingness to cooperate may contribute to the success of your surgery. Fear and negativity may work against the process.
- Restrict your visitors and phone calls. Give yourself time to heal.
- Be sure and communicate your needs and concerns to the doctors and nurses around you. They are there to help.
- Talk to your health care providers about getting patient support, such as having a cancer survivor contact you. Some resources are listed in the last chapter of this book.

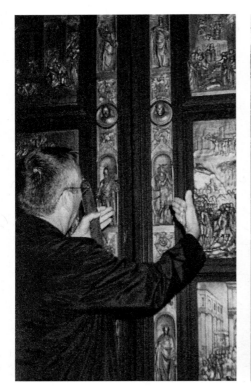 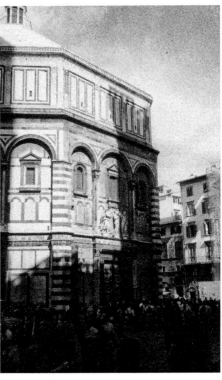

Ghiberti's panels are on the Baptistery's east doors, bronzed with lustrous hues, and depicting inspirational stories. The Baptistery was consecrated in the 12th century.

CHAPTER SEVEN

Recovery From Surgery:
Reconstruction and Ghiberti's Panels

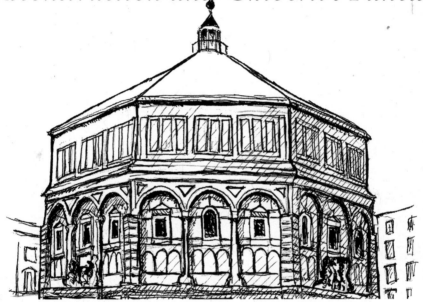

T he original church in Florence's Cathedral Square is the Baptistery, an eight-sided structure standing by itself like a defiant monument to the past. Built in the 5th century, it was reconstructed in the 12th century and is still being used as a place of worship. The geometric patterns on its exterior and mosaic designs in its dome reveal the Germanic and Eastern influence of the early Roman Empire. The Baptistery seems out of place with the rest of the architecture we've been seeing in Italy. Proud and unique, it seems to be holding its chin up as if to say, "Look at me. I've been through it all and I'm still here."

Today, the Baptistery is renowned for ten bronze-covered panels on its east doors depicting scenes from the Bible. Just like the church, these panels have been rebuilt, replicas of work by Lorenzo Ghiberti in 1425 A.D. I am trying to see them as a peasant might have viewed them during the Early Renaissance. In a world in which the printed word was not available to all, and mass communication was more than 500 years away, the church used these panels to depict stories from the Bible. They were a table of contents to the Old Testament.

I step back from these panels and think about the stories I would be telling someday of my cancer experience. In a similar way, I would be sculpturing them like a Ghiberti door, selecting only specific scenes as a way to give meaning to the event, and superficially bronzing them with lustrous hues of memory as I preserve them. I make a mental note to pay attention to balance, perspective, and realism if I want to replicate these stories artfully. The negative and positive aspects of the ordeal need to be kept in balance; the perspective needs to be multi-dimensional; and the memoir needs to reflect reality.

The First Six Weeks After Surgery

When I came home from the hospital, I went through a period of elation, a quiet and stillness that only someone worn down by the strife of reconstruction can appreciate; a relief from the onslaught of harsh treatments, a newly acquired appreciation of the ordinary rituals of life, awakening to a day free of doctor appointments and hospital schedules, relishing the taste of food again and focusing on concerns other than disease. I knew it was just a temporary respite, however. Completing the rest of chemotherapy was looming in the distance.

My first week after returning home was a blur to me. I was well supplied with pain pills and glad to get out of the hospital. I took time to look out onto our trees in the back yard and marveled we were already in the last weeks of May. By the second week, the pain pills were playing havoc with my stomach, and I decided it was time to stop taking them. I switched to Tylenol and sleeping pills for a few days, and then decided I could get by just taking the Tylenol. Cards, phone calls, and visits from friends kept me in good spirits, but I would occasionally wake up in the middle of the night, anxious, and still sore from the operation.

One night, I woke up and couldn't get back to sleep. I got up, walked into a dimly lit bathroom, reached for the shelf where we kept all of our medicines in a container, fuzzily took out one of my sleeping pills, swallowed it, and then went back to bed.

Shortly thereafter, I felt like hot liquid was being pumped through my veins in double time. My heart was racing so much I was alarmed. I woke my husband.

"Something's wrong. I took a sleeping pill and I feel like I'm on fire."

"That's strange," he pondered. "Did you have any reaction before?"

"No. I don't get it." My voice was shaky. "We better call the doctor."

He got up to see what the problem was.

"Where's the pill bottle? See if it lists any side effects."

This time, I put on my glasses and turned on the light. With utter dismay, I realized I had grabbed the wrong bottle, a cold medication loaded with Benzedrine that had been prescribed for my husband, David Larson, not me, "Carol Larson." Fortunately, we kept an information sheet on all the side effects of this particular pill, and they were not grave.

I shook my head with relief. Dave, sure the drug would wear off in a couple of hours, went back to sleep.

That was at 3:00 a.m. By 9:00 that morning, I had read John Grisham's book "The Street Lawyer" and still felt like I was on medication. All day, I was wide awake, nervous, and jittery. I watched two movies during the day that failed to put me to sleep. Finally, that night I "crashed."

This was a substantial lesson to me of the foolhardiness of keeping left-over medication in the house. The real mistake was that I needed to look more closely at what I was choosing. As a good friend advised me later, "Next time, put on your stupid glasses."

My stitches were healing nicely, and the new ostomy wasn't giving me any problems. I thought of it in my recovery as a minor impediment, a minor detour while my main thoroughfare was being repaired. However, by the end of the fourth week after surgery, I was surprised that I was still having so much rectal discomfort. I couldn't be on my feet for more than 20 minutes without hurting. I had to lie down in the back seat of our car if we were going to ride for more than an hour. I felt phantom pains that made me have the urge to evacuate. I was especially getting impatient to feel better as Laura's wedding approached, just one month away. I felt I needed to do something to speed up my healing for my daughter's wedding.

I decided to turn to an acupuncturist to help me with my pain management with the approval of my colorectal surgeon. Where I goofed was that I did not follow a regular referral process. I had heard of this "fabulous" acupuncturist from a friend of mine, so I made a decision I would pay the money out of pocket to go to this particular person at another location.

In retrospect, I should have paid attention to two red flags when turning to an alternative therapy. Although the beginning sessions were not too steep, the mounting costs for continuing her care would have been considerable; and two, her credentials were questionable. Still, I reasoned, she must be all right. After all, my friend had been pleased (of course, she was not treating him for cancer).

The first visit started out soothing with music and candles surrounding me as I lay down on a white sheeted examining table. The acupuncturist examined my tongue and deemed me essentially healthy. I ignored a strong suggestion to buy into the herbs sold on the side. As she started the process of acupuncture, however, some of her methods made me question the wisdom of what I was doing. I could hardly feel the pricks, but she was poking her needles on the skin above my anal area of my body not too far from my surgery. I thought she was going to place them in my head, or even in my feet. It did not hurt, but I felt this was a risky thing for her to be doing.

My pain felt somewhat abated, so I was willing to go back. What did I know? Maybe that's the way things were done. After the second session, however, I realized she was stimulating nerves that were better to be numbed in an area of my body that was no longer being used. I came home feeling pronounced pain.

I called my colorectal surgeon, asking for some advice. He seemed perplexed until he asked me to describe my treatment and where she placed the needles. After I told him, there was a distinct, "What?" that had a thud to it.

"She did what? How could you let her do that to you?" he asked.

I gulped. I didn't have a good answer to that one. "Well, I've never gone to an acupuncturist before. I didn't know what to expect. Didn't you say it was okay?"

"I never thought she would operate so close to my surgery," he countered. "Is she a doctor? How did you get her name?"

"I think so, but I don't know." I stammered. "My friend has been going to her for years for a back problem."

"Does she know anything about colorectal cancer?"

At that point, I felt all I was doing was giving lame excuses to the sheriff for making a wrong turn.

"Probably not," I admitted. "I explained to her I had an ileostomy and was no longer using my colon, but even at the time I was wondering if she was grasping the implications of what I was telling her. I should've been less trusting, I guess."

He told me I would have to come in if the pain increased, but thank goodness, it diminished. I may have extended my recovery, but I did eventually get better.

By the time we were getting ready for Laura's wedding, the episode became a minor mishap, but it remained a lesson for me about the seriousness of turning to unauthorized sources for questionable treatments.

Alternative methods of healing, certainly, can be effective and soothing, but the Latin *caveat emptor* "buyer beware" should be included in that statement. No doubt that there is strong mind/body connection in healing. Acupuncture and biofeedback have been proven methods of relieving pain. Just because they're labeled "alternative" and "natural" does not mean they are harmless, however. One thing I could have done to protect myself would be to go to an acupuncturist that would have been in touch with my doctors. Or call my doctor as soon as I had some questions. I could have also gone to the Internet site www.quackwatch.org and used that as a guide in making intelligent decisions.

Psalms — Songs of Praise

Just one week before the wedding, a harsh windstorm swept its way through our community and toppled our 80 year old elm tree onto our back yard. When I woke up in the morning and looked out, all I could see was destruction. We had been trying to get ready for out-of-town guests and a Sunday brunch for our new in-laws. Now all that seemed impossible.

"It'll cost us at least $1,000 to have that tree removed," Dave lamented.

On top of our hospital and wedding bills, that was disturbing news. The world seemed against us at that point. I fell into a slump and went back to bed. I started to doubt that I would even have the strength to go through with Laura's wedding, which we had been anticipating with so much pleasure. Later, in the afternoon, Dave and I sat in our kitchen writing down numbers for a tree removal service that would be able to come out during the week. We were pretty skeptical. The storm had hit our whole area hard, and there would be numerous requests for help.

I heard some noise outside and I went to the window. Looking down from the second story of our house, I will never forget the scene below. There, sawing and toting branches, were more than twenty of our neighbors, adults, teenagers, and older children, coming together to clean up our back yard because they were good Samaritans. They had heard of my cancer ordeal, and knew that our daughter was going to be getting married soon.

How could you have a bad perspective when there was so much goodness in people? Dave went down to help them and I brought out cookies and lemonade. There was so much camaraderie and good-natured laughter, it was like a party, but through it all, they worked all afternoon. By dusk, our lawn was in good shape once again.

Cancer can't destroy kindness or the joy of a wedding. Our daughter Laura and Scott were married the next week. I know I am biased, but Laura really was a beautiful bride. My granddaughter Courtney decided at the last minute not to come down the aisle, but she still thought of herself as the flower girl. What I didn't expect was that Laura had selected the soloist to sing "Eagle's Wings." In the program, she requested the whole congregation to join together singing the refrain. I was choked up with emotion as I heard them sing,

> "And he will raise you up on eagle's wings,
> Bear you on the breath of dawn,
> Make you to shine in the sun,
> And hold you in the palm of his hand."

They were singing to Laura and Scott, but I felt they were singing to David and me as well, giving us their blessings by this song, and glorifying the power of faith over adversity.

Radiation Proctitis

One decision I had to make before starting chemotherapy was the timing of my ileostomy reversal. After the fiasco with the acupuncturist, and having some unusually harsh reactions to some follow-up tests, it became clear that I had developed a condition called "radiation proctitis." This is a condition caused by damage to the lining of the rectum from radiation, which can occur at any time, from months to years after a patient is done with radiation.

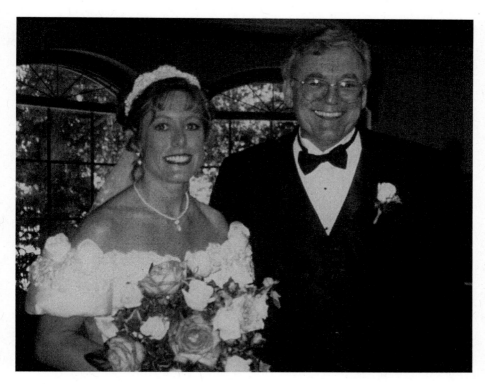

Laura and Dave before the wedding.

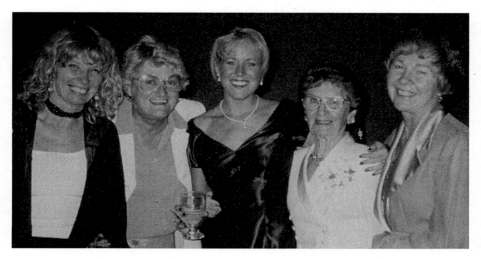

Meg, Cookie, Jennifer, Jean, and me at the reception.

This is quite common and usually it is short lived. This complicated matters in that the proctitis was severe in my case, causing additional post surgical pain and bleeding.

I decided to wait to have my "take down" until I was finished with treatments. Most of my rectum had been removed, and without much of a holding tank, control would be an adjustment for a while. One of the probable side effects of having chemo would most likely be diarrhea. I figured, to put it bluntly, a reversal of my ileostomy at this point would be a big pain in the butt. Instead, we agreed I would come in at intervals to be dilated to prevent the colon from closing up. In retrospect, this was a very wise decision. Because of the way things turned out for me, it would've been a disaster if I had decided to have my reversal at that point.

Support Groups

I tried to prepare myself for this ordeal by going to two different support groups. Both of them were composed of people with different kinds of cancer, at different stages.

The first one was like a rap group, with many people who were dealing with more advanced stages of cancer. The focus of the group was directed to one gentleman who had just been told he wouldn't be given any more chemotherapy. Obviously his situation was dire. As I introduced myself and told the group I was just going to begin my major treatments, my concerns were dwarfed by the severity of what this other gentleman was facing. I felt sorry for him, but also felt short-changed, because I needed help as well. I never went back, realizing with humility and gratitude that I was misplaced in that group, lucky to be at the stage that I was.

The other support group I attended was a general meeting where we heard about common issues cancer patients might face. Sponsored by the American Cancer Society the speakers knew what they were talking about, having been cancer patients. Their stories were touching and inspiring. The only drawbacks to this group were that the sessions were given to a larger audience of about 50 people, and held few and far between. I needed something more ongoing and more personal, a group for patients who had colorectal cancer.

My Ghiberti Panels of Courageous Friends

Some of my closest friends are real life heroes. Their stories provided me with inspiration and guidance giving me strength to face chemotherapy.

Mary Lou and I have lived through each crisis of our lives together since 8th grade. When her first husband, Darryl, was diagnosed with cancer in his early '30s, I remembered their tremendous courage. At a key moment when I was down, Darryl called and reminded me, "This too, shall pass." I needed to hear those words.

There have been other friends from high school who have had to contend with various types of cancer. Barb, Sharon, Joe, Marlys, Gordy's brother, and JoEllen deserve a bronzed door for bravely facing excruciating ordeals for years until cancer finally took their lives. My dear Athena has superbly lived with the threat of lymphoma. Claire's son underwent chemotherapy and is, at this point, cancer free. Looking to the past, Nancy, Jean, and Darlene (John's wife) overcame breast cancer. Bev's husband, Al and other dear friends, like Paul and Stan, have also had to deal with cancer. Pat B. survived cancer. Andy did not. So many people from my ostomy group (OAMA) like Sue and Karen B. have survived recurrences. There is hardly anyone we know whose families have not had some kind of life-threatening disease, and yet they maintained their humanity and their sense of humor.

Two of Red's closest friends, Dana and Gary, who were like brothers to me, overcame life-threatening situations and continued to lead vital lives. When Dana was 17, he survived a diving accident leaving him a quadriplegic. He finished school, became a gifted writer and managed two apartment buildings. He found a loving relationship and established a new life with Rozanne, also in a wheelchair. They taught me to make the most of what you have. Dana died two years before my diagnosis, but their determination and humor remained with me all through my ordeals.

Gary suffered a stroke in his late 50's which, according to one doctor, would be life-limiting. With the help of his exceptionally supportive wife, Maria, he overcame the stroke moving on to a miraculous recovery. He returned to making furniture, and leading a good life. Dick, who hosted our Christmas party every year, succumbed to mortal effects of a stroke. Anita's husband, Roger, died in his sleep when they were in their 30s, and she went on to do an excellent job raising their family.

And then there was my friend Barb, who had been diagnosed with Lou Gehrig's disease just about the same time I was diagnosed with colorectal cancer. Two neurologists predicted that by summer she would no longer have the strength to ever walk again. With determination, she put herself on the best health regimen possible, never giving up. Years later, like a miracle, her symptoms almost completely disappeared but the emotional battles she overcame demonstrated to me the power of a positive attitude.

**Tips for Travelers After Having Surgery:

- Follow all post-operative directions. Call your doctor if you have any questions.
- Your body has been through a lot. Give yourself plenty of time to rest and recuperate. Enjoy the good times.
- Discard any unused medicines from your hospital stay. Always read the labels carefully before taking any pills.
- Alternative methods of healing can be beneficial but check out the credentials and costs of anyone administering therapy. Make sure that there is two-way communication between your practitioner and your doctors.
- Join a support group. Turn to supportive friends and family. If there is no colorectal cancer support group in your area, see Resources in the back of this book.
- Think of heroes you have known and what can be learned from them.

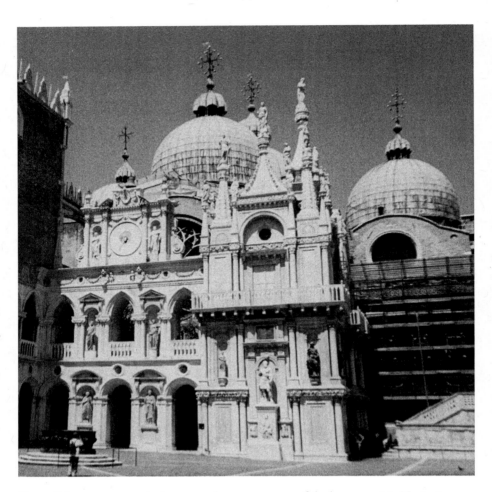

Doges Palace represents the beauty and empowerment of the human spirit. Venice is an amazing tribute to survival regardless of adversity.

CHAPTER EIGHT

Chemotherapy:
Venice and Trying to Stay Afloat

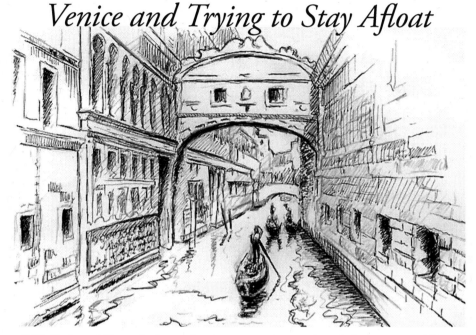

L ife is a delicate balance between preservation and destruction. Venice
flourished because its people created a beautiful refuge from barbarians
on islands in a lagoon. It is decaying because of the ravages the water
has wreaked on its remains. Based on 117 islands, spanned by 400 bridges,
and intersected by 150 canals, it is sinking at the rate of two inches per
decade, but it is still the best preserved medieval city in Europe. It is a tribute
to survival in spite of adversity.

At the heart of Venice is St. Mark's Square. Making our way through the
pigeons, we take pictures of its ornate cathedral. We then proceed to Doge's
Palace where, once inside, we marvel at the gilded ceiling and walls meant as
a display of the power of the Venetian Republic that ruled Venice for 400
years. The Doges government left a legacy of elegance.

There was a downside to this splendor, however. We descend steep stairs
in a narrow, crude passageway to cells where prisoners were shackled and
held down. We look up through barred windows to see the famous "Bridge
of Sighs" where the condemned criminals of later years crossed over to the

prison. Thankful to leave these bleak surroundings, we climb the stairs back to the opulence of the main room.

This palace seems to represent the beauty and empowerment of the human spirit; the prison evokes feelings of despondency, when depression suppresses all life-giving powers.

We walk, en masse, around the palace with other passengers on our tour. Marco, a handsome man who appears to be in his sixties, has a wife who hangs onto his arm wherever they go. Her possessiveness makes us wary. When we are waiting to use the women's restroom, however, she turns to me in an extremely nervous state and inquires, "Do you know where my husband is? I've lost him." In a flash, I realize that she has been holding onto him for dear life. I explain to her where we are, that she is safe, and I will be waiting for her after she comes out of the bathroom. A few minutes later, I look around and she is nowhere to be found. I look up the stairs and discover one of our younger female companions leading her by the hand. Nice.

Marco's wife reminds me of myself, another reminder of how fragile we all can be. I remember how that feels because I have been there too, when I was dealing my own feelings of isolation, confusion, and worry during chemotherapy. They were the worst emotions I had to encounter. Sickness and discomfort were easier for me to handle, by comparison. The sound of a reassuring voice, a human touch, and the knowledge that other people were watching over me were by far the most powerful antidotes against the destruction of my spirit. This was a time in my life when I most fully realized how much the help of other people could keep me from sinking.

Returning to Chemotherapy

At the end of July following the wedding, I was supposed to resume my chemotherapy sessions in earnest, coming in once a week for six weeks with two weeks of vacation in between cycles. By this time, I was becoming familiar with the maze of Medicine Land. I knew my way around and was more skilled in expressing my needs in an effective way.

I was taking a proactive role in my health care and learning to speak a new language that would improve my communication with both doctors and nurses.

Totally unexpected was the fact that my most supportive group in regard to my health were my doctors, nurses and other patients. I was welcomed back to chemotherapy like a returning traveler. It was usually an upbeat and positive experience going in for treatments.

"How was the wedding?" The oncologist asked me.

The nurses wanted to know, "Did you bring any pictures?"

When I entered the room to get my dose of chemo, olive green Naugahyde lounging chairs were well occupied with other people like me, coming in for prescribed dosages of whatever type of chemo was needed. The conversations were frequently chatty; we talked about the latest book or the hottest movie in the theaters. There was joking and catching up with the news of the week; unbelievably, there were few complaints about the needles attached to our veins.

Some people who were going to be there for hours watched videos while others slept. It turned out one of my favorite nurses had a boy in Laura's kindergarten class. Another beautiful nurse and I swapped stories that made us laugh. Nobody dwelt on the negative or went overboard with too much sympathy. Even when I finished a series of blood tests walking out with three bandages on my arm, my oncologist came by and remarked, "Looks like you got in a fight with a cat."

The Chemotherapy Canal

At first, going through chemotherapy seemed like a gondola ride. I would go in for my treatments, knowing that competent people were steering the course. If I had a day or two when I felt slightly under the weather, I would just lie back and enjoy the scenery. The majority of the week I felt almost like my old self. On those days, I would play a few rounds of golf with the assistance of a cart, or meet my friends for lunch or dinner.

I didn't fully realize until I had cancer how easy my life was, being blessed with good health and abundant energy. I was used to a luxurious stream of comfort. I never knew how quickly the current could change. People go through chemotherapy with variant levels of difficulty. Having an ileostomy complicated my responses to treatments, but, as I found out later, some of the problems I encountered could have been avoided.

By the middle of August, it was if my gondola was sandbagged by unexpected cargo, making it harder for me to keep my balance. I no longer could just be a passive passenger. I needed to make adjustments just to keep my equilibrium. This required problem solving.

My oncologist monitored my blood levels, observed my stamina, and was on the outlook for any severe depression or tiredness, but I realized I needed to do my part if I wanted to weather the designated distance with the least damage done.

For me, it was a wise decision not to have my ileostomy reversed until after the chemotherapy was over. I was having daily bouts with diarrhea, but was only aware of it because of slight cramping and the contents of my bag. I felt like I had a constant flu, becoming progressively dehydrated. I was told to keep drinking water, but that was hard to do once I was nauseated. My blood count dropped, so they gave me two hours of intravenous fluids and skipped that week of chemotherapy. A few days later, I lay in bed for hours that week just trying to be still so I could get some relief from cramps, which were becoming more pronounced. I always thought of myself as a person who had a zest for life. There I was, listless, enduring pain and not knowing what to do.

I decided to call my oncologist, and was given a prescription for an anti-diarrhetic drug. Like magic, the pain disappeared. I didn't realize that even though I had an ileostomy, I could get help with the discomfort of diarrhea, just like anyone else. From that point on, I took the anti-diarrhetic drug regularly, which helped me immensely. My first real problem had been solved, and I was strongly back on course.

Nausea was my next, most immediate problem. When I reached my first break at the end of August, I almost cancelled. Once again, I called the doctor's office and got a prescription for an anti-nausea pill. I wanted to say *grazie* – thankful for feeling better.

With these medications in my luggage, Dave and I, Red and Sandy left for a townhouse on the North Shore. My brother invented games we could play even though my energy was low, like racing each other on pinball machines and playing makeshift miniature golf on a deserted track of land. We took 30 mile road trips up to Grand Marais and bought chocolate sodas, which strangely enough appealed to my sluggish appetite. I came back from my vacation strengthened by rest and determined to go through my second cycle better than I did before. So far, so good.

Things That Helped

By the middle of September, I was struggling with distaste for most food and tiredness for much of the week. Although my white cell blood count was low, my neutrophils were good, so I didn't have to skip any more treatments. Neutrophils are specialized white cells that fight infections. By now I knew that problematic blood cell counts were not unexpected. It only meant the chemo was working, at least on healthy cells (hopefully, if there were any residual bad ones, it was taking care of those too).

I tracked my progress just like my oncologist was doing, finding it helpful to keep a journal to identify predictable patterns. Even this abnormal life had a rhythm to it. Resting for a day or two after each treatment helped me to restore reserves of energy. When good days came, I did the things I most enjoyed doing. This included going into school and volunteering my services for a couple of hours. I missed the fun and excitement of work and was looking forward to going back to a full time job. Retirement was not for me. Not just yet.

Usually by the weekends, I felt better. My sister's family visited me from California, and we finished crossword puzzles on my deck, watched videos, and took short walks in the afternoon. I tried to get together with friends whenever possible. It took an effort on my part to partake in these activities, but they were distracting and helped raise my morale.

I managed to avoid mouth sores, a common side effect. I believe that the fluoride treatment my dentist gave me, previous to starting chemo, gets credit for this. He also encouraged me to use a non-alcoholic toothpaste because he predicted the regular kind would've been too irritating.

My appetite for sex, just like my appetite for food, diminished temporarily. My need for tenderness and love hadn't changed. Oddly enough, some times I felt very happy, I guess because people were so good to me. That made up for a lot of things I lacked. The random acts of kindness that people bestowed on me held me up. Letters and cards sustained me. I read them over and over again, even the ones from just good acquaintances, experiencing plenty of Hallmark moments that would've made good commercials.

Phone calls were like lifelines. Cookie would call regularly from Escondido, California. My cousin Meg called me each week from San Francisco giving me inspiration and support.

"It's important that you live in the present," Meg advised. "Let love and energy flow into your consciousness." I smiled at that statement, because it sounded so much like California, but it actually helped me focus my energy on healing. Looking ahead too far into the future caused me to be more anxious. She sent me some inspirational tapes I could listen to while resting and I did more soul searching than I have ever done before. I prayed a lot and found solace in a renewed spirituality.

My Bridge of Sighs

I managed well until October, and then my whole body bogged down. The anti-diarrhetic drugs were not doing their job anymore. Going downstairs to put in a load of wash in was a major undertaking. I stopped going over to school. I couldn't seem to maintain food in my system for long and I lost my appetite entirely. Even water was repugnant. I rarely got sick, but was nauseated most of the time. Hamburger was like rubber and bread tasted like sawdust. Getting adequate nutrition was becoming a problem without me even realizing it; my throat was dry most of the time. Well meaning people would keep pushing food in front of me, but that just seemed to make it worse. I was progressively having more difficulty swallowing, so I resorted to ice cream and yogurt malts. Anything chocolate and creamy was appealing to me. Fortified prepared liquid food would have helped my nutritional needs, but I gagged when I tried to get it down.

Maybe because of the stress, I found I was confused at times and finding it hard to concentrate. People who have been there call it "chemo-brain." I've never read any research on this phenomenon, but I experienced it. I began feeling separated from the people, sort of like I was invaded by The Body Snatchers. Dave and my children took over all of the household duties. Every day was a struggle to overcome depression, but sometimes it was a relief just to go with the sorrow that I was feeling. The trouble was if I stayed too long with my negative thoughts, they just seemed to weigh me down further. More and more, I felt as if I was sinking, heading for a whirlpool I wanted to avoid.

It was just a matter of time before the diarrhea and my lack of a proper diet would cause my body to rebel. I spent one morning at the hospital with a partial blockage. The food I was forcing myself to eat was not digesting as it should. Vicki lavaged me (injected my intestine with water) but it was necessary for me to go on a liquid diet for the next day.

Later that week, I went in to see another oncologist, rather than my regular doctor. She was so alarmed by all the weight I'd been losing (a total of 25 pounds since I started treatment) that she almost wouldn't begin my second cycle of chemotherapy. I pleaded with her that I was only about half done with my treatments and I didn't think I could stand to prolong it longer. She did a double take.

"Where did you get that idea? It says here five months. I think you'll be done by Christmas."

I realized at that moment I forgot to add my treatments before surgery. I needed five months, not five cycles composed of six weeks.

"Really? Christmas?" I asked her like a child realizing there really was a Santa.

Wryly she remarked, "If I'm wrong, I'm going to ask someone else to call you back."

I was given another treatment, only this time, I gagged, and almost couldn't go through with it. I went home extremely motivated to gain weight, but it was harder than I thought. I had to force myself to eat anything at all. I couldn't figure this out .Why was I so nauseated? I started to lose my will to complete chemotherapy, even until December. It was my daughter Jenny who came through with a solution.

Major Sustenance

Friday night, Dave and I took Jenny to dinner. When the food arrived, I had such revulsion to it, I told them I was ready to give up taking any more treatments. My daughter listened very carefully to what I was saying and remarked, "You know, Mom, your symptoms sound just like some of the athletes I coached. Dry mouth, inability to swallow, and nausea. Those are all signs of dehydration. Could that be your problem?"

"No," I said with certainty. "I drink at least eight glasses of water a day."

Dave corrected me, "But you really don't."

I tried to protest, but he came back with, "You pour yourself eight glasses a day, but I've been watching you, and you only drink a little of each glass before you pour it down the sink."

I realized, at that moment, that what he was saying was true.

Jenny added, "Dehydration can make you nauseous and very sick, Mom. It's serious."

That made sense to me. I was probably dehydrated. The diarrhea from chemotherapy can cause this, and I remember reading that a person with an ileostomy was even more susceptible to this condition. On this assumption, I drank a cup of cocoa and glasses of water throughout the night. By the next morning, I experienced a transformation. I was no longer as nauseous. I began to eat some real food.

As soon as I felt better, my old optimism returned. I did get a call the next morning telling me that it was confirmed: I would be done by mid-December, even earlier than Christmas. I was overjoyed!

I finished the last two treatments in mid-October doing much better. I still kept taking anti-diarrhetic drugs, but I was drinking at least eight glasses of water a day. My appetite was poor, but at least I could make myself ingest food better than before. I was still having troubling swallowing. I was drinking soups or hot fudge yogurt malts, so my nutritional needs were lacking. Nevertheless, I managed to gain a few pound eating this way, and my oncologist was pleased by my progress.

S.O.S. — Calls for Help

Unfortunately, I was weaker than I thought. After my last chemo treatment in this cycle, I went in to have my colon dilated, trying to get ready for my January reversal of my ileostomy. The dilation went well, but the radiation proctitis had worsened causing me to bleed quite a bit after I came home. I became very cold. My daughter Tami talked to me on the phone, and was alarmed my speech seemed so sluggish. Tami's sharp instincts took over and she immediately drove over to our house. My hands were bluish, my face terribly drained of color, and I couldn't stop shivering, so she loaded me up with blankets, a heater, warm socks, and liquids. My heart was pounding by this point. Finally, she just held me, and was ready to call the doctor, when I settled down. Two hours later, I was much better. I went through a couple of uncomfortable days, but finally, by the end of the week, I seemed to be improving.

Meg flew in and stayed with us over the weekend. She was going to go to a daytime retreat near our area, and wanted a quiet, restful place at night. At 3:00 a.m., I woke up in excruciating pain. My stomach felt like a cement wall. I took some pain pills and mercifully fell asleep. The next morning, however, I was in agony. Dave needed to work, so my daughter Laura drove over to our house. We called Vicki who said I better see her immediately.

With all this commotion, and even though I would have spasms of pain that took my breath away, I looked over at my cousin and remarked, "Hey, Meg. Aren't you glad you've selected such a quiet, restful place to stay?"

By the time Laura drove me to the hospital, my stomach was totally rejecting food, and I was vomiting. Vicki took me down in a wheelchair to the emergency room. The Admittance clerk seemed to be annoyed when she saw us, and questioned if we really had to be there, because in between pains, I didn't look like I was sick. When I started to have dry heaves in the waiting room, however, they rolled me to the emergency room fast. After a couple of X-rays, determining a blockage, I was blessedly given morphine for the pain, and hooked up to an IV machine. They then admitted me to the hospital.

It took me almost a full day afterward for my system to unblock and to start tolerating liquids and a little bit of humor. The next day, my oncologist visited me in the hospital. The last time I saw him I was doing fairly well. When he walked into the room he shook his head and said, "I can't leave you alone for a minute and you get into trouble."

On the second night, at 3:00 a.m., I woke up with more cramping. The nurse called the doctor and got a prescription for stronger pain medication. She came in and sympathetically told me I would have to wait a half hour before she could give it to me. I told her I was just grateful that it was coming. Then she sat down with me and started to ask questions about my children, my job, and what I had gone through so far with my cancer treatment. Before I knew it, the half hour was up and I got more relief. I'll never forget how kind she was in doing this. Another wonderful nurse. Another random act of kindness.

By the third day, I'd had it. In the wake of all this misery, I was feeling depressed and overwhelmed. More tests were ordered which I had to complete, one of which was a stomach X-ray. I feared this test in that they needed to basically put a miniature camera down my throat, which played out in my mind as horrendous. I was wheeled back down to the X-ray department, and into the hall. Scared of having more pain, I lay there waiting for more than an hour, feeling lost, confused, and worried. Out of all my experiences, I think this was the worst. I lost my sense of self. It seemed to me nothing was ever going to get any better. I felt submerged.

Finally, the doctor came over to me and she apologized. An elderly woman had come in on an emergency, and they had needed to take care of her first. Could I forgive them for making me wait so long? They would take me in just one more half hour. Everything would be O.K. No, the test would not be painful.

Immediately, with that reassurance, I felt a surge of relief. This one act of consideration was all I needed to restore my confidence. I still counted. It would be all right. I gave myself a small lecture about making this situation more dramatic than it had to be. I directed my attention to a team of nurses down the hall from me, talking about their day. The camaraderie, the ease of conversation, and the sense of belonging were reminiscent of my job at school, or any job, where workers are compatible with one another. A doctor came up to them, cracked a joke, and they all laughed. Some day, I vowed, if I ever got another chance, I'd find myself some fun place to work again.

When they were ready for me, I was given a mild sedative, and my throat was sprayed to make the camera slip down easier. This was supposed to be the worst part of the test, but I was puzzled to find out how good it felt to have my throat numb. I was given the results immediately. I had small ulcers, which they would be taken care of with medication. On top of that, they discovered I had a yeast infection in my throat, a product of malnutrition and dryness, which explained why it had been so hard for me to swallow foods. Both were easily fixable. Then they wheeled me back to my room.

I stayed with the IV machine two more days. My body was shot, my hemoglobin, my white blood cell count, and potassium level were low, and so they kept me for six days until my condition improved. I had to go through three more tests before I left the hospital, but the good news was that they found no cancer. I was extremely weak, and lost five more pounds, so that was discouraging. It was so unfair. I was supposed to be on my "break". That seemed to be what was happening to me. I felt I was breaking down.

I finally was allowed to go home, but by now, I lost my faith in my recuperative powers. The problem was Dave had to go back to work that day, and I realized after he left, I was afraid to be left alone. I phoned Meg's mom, my Aunt Jean, and she came running over with a hot fudge sundae. I ate the whole thing. Gradually, I began to regain my optimism and by the end of the day I went from feeling fearful to euphoric. I realized I had turned the corner and I just had a little bit more distance to go before I would be on safe shores once again.

This is when I started earnestly to improve my nutrition, get more exercise, and take regular naps every day. Gradually I became stronger in body and in spirit.

But I didn't do it all alone. It was sometimes hard for me to accept help from other people, but that's what I did. Dave continued to drive me to the rest of my treatments. My daughters took turns cleaning our house. My brother, Red, suggested I take this time to write a biography of my mom. My sister and friends wrote me wonderful letters. Some of my friends apologized for sharing some of their problems with me at this time, but the truth of the matter was that I needed to think about other things, not just my own struggle with cancer. It was important for me to feel a part of life and to be able to help others too, as much as I could.

I learned two important lessons from this experience: There are many things a patient can do to minimize devastating side effects of chemotherapy, and there is nothing quite as restorative as the help of others when life gets scary and overwhelming.

**Tips for Travelers Going Through Chemotherapy:

- Focus on the present. Let go of minor problems. Live as well as you can.
- Be kind to yourself.
- Let the kindness of others help to buoy you up.
- Enhance your life with peace.
- Faith, spirituality, meditation, deep breathing, and imagery are ways to get there.
- Express your emotions. Cultivate the ones that encourage you to heal.
- Clearly communicate your symptoms to your oncologist. Do not assume that just because you are going through chemotherapy you have to be sick. There is effective medicine to help side effects.
- Track your progress in a journal. Not only is this therapeutic, but you may be able to identify helpful, predictable patterns.
- Do as much as you can to preserve your health. A dentist knowledgeable about cancer can give you help for preventative measures against mouth sores. Make sure you are getting enough nutrition in your diet. Dehydration can become a problem. Take seriously the suggestion that you should drink at least eight glasses of water a day
- Don't forget these three R's:
    REST especially right after each treatment.
    RELAX by doing the things you most enjoy.
    REACH OUT and stay involved with other people. Accept and appreciate their help

*****Someday, you can pass on what you have learned to someone else.

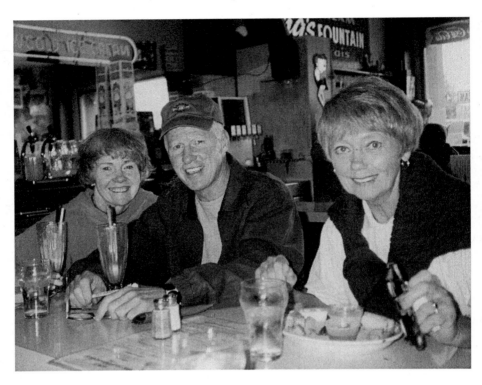

Me, Red, and Sandy on my first break from chemotherapy.

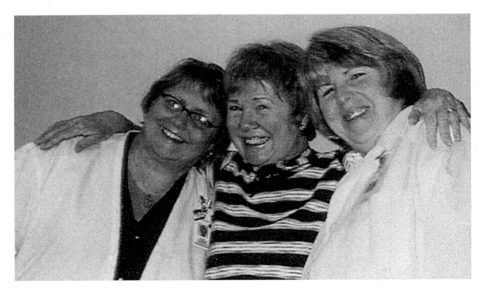

Vicki and Julie. Enterostomal nurses can be a great source of support.

CHAPTER NINE

Areas of Combat:
The Gladiators

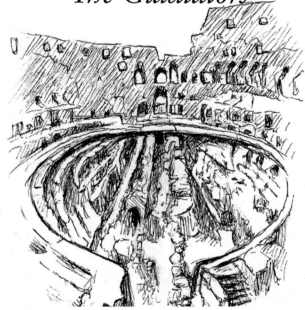

What does it mean to "put up a good fight?" The Coliseum in Rome, constructed in 80 A.D., addressed this question for its participants, a theater designated for the ultimate reality show of its time. At its peak, it could seat 50,000 people. Four stories high, there were nets along the sides to protect the spectators as they watched gladiators bludgeon their foes to survive. It's hard to escape the gore of this place, nor forget the bloody encounters violently on display mostly at the expense of slaves, prisoners, and Christians.

Gladiators were summoned to their fate when we looked at the ruins of underground passages leading to the main floor of the arena. With its cruelty and viciousness, this was hardly an admirable "sport." If the gladiator fought well, the crowd would cheer and perhaps intercede with a "thumbs up", giving him or her a reprieve to come back and fight another day. (Women were gladiators too.) Even so, putting up an undaunted effort would not save gladiators if the Caesar or the spectators decided arbitrarily to give them a "thumbs down." Their lives would be ended. It all depended on the whims of the moment. Gladiators faced up to the basic questions of life and death.

I think about the widespread belief that those of us who have cancer are supposed to be on the order of gladiators and advised to put up a good "fight" against this disease. We are, of course, up against an internal rampage of cancer cells within our body, rather than an external enemy, but aren't we also facing up to the questions of life and death?

There are problems with that analogy. This is not a game, nor are we engaged in an act of hostility. The word "fight" is appropriate only in the sense of rallying determination, resisting losing hope, making ourselves strong, learning all we can about what we have to face, and adapting a mental attitude of being the victor, and not the victim. Anger will not destroy the cancer cells within us, but establishing a peaceful state of mind will make our efforts easier to bear.

Just like the gladiators, no matter how courageously we fight, people who have cancer may not be given a "thumbs up" in the struggle to survive. The most valiant heroes aren't always successful overcoming cancer and should not be made to feel they are to blame if, despite their efforts, they are given a "thumbs down" and cancer overtakes their bodies. The reality is that we are all struggling to find our way through our maze of underground passages trying to reach the best arena of life we can find while we are alive.

I think back to my last days in the arena fending off harsh side effects of my treatments. Even a warrior gets weary with continued onslaughts. When a person gets to this point, "winning" is making the most of life, no matter what the outcome. This is not a bloody battle to be fought, but a quest to live life making every day count. That is the victory.

Reversal of a Decision

As I was nearing the end of my treatments, I had another appointment with the colorectal surgeon for a final dilation before my ileostomy would be reversed. I was dreading this process, which had become progressively more painful. The proctitis had weakened the lining of my rectum and augmented the pain of any intrusive test. Heavy bleeding after any rectal exam had become a regular occurrence.

Two days before my visit, the surgeon's receptionist called me and I was told just to come in for a consultation. This was an unusual summons. I fearfully pondered what the colorectal surgeon might want to tell me. When I came into his office, I could see dismay was written all over his face.

"I'm sorry," he began, "but I'm having problems advocating the prospect of reversing your ileostomy."

I started to cry. A silent voice within me was protesting.

"Only 5% patients have severe chronic proctitis," he continued, "and you are one of them."

"Do you mean you think I should wait?" I asked feebly, hoping this was what he meant, but really, knowing it was not.

He measured his words so there would be no misunderstanding.

"No. The damage to what's left of your rectum is irreversible. It probably won't be getting much better than it is now."

For almost a minute, I couldn't speak. He finally said, "You might want to consider keeping the ileostomy permanent, unless you are willing to go through much suffering to try to do without it."

I know my voice was shaky when I tried to protest. "If I could endure the pain, would my bodily functions eventually return to normal?"

"Even in the most ideal situation, after having most of your rectum removed, you would be battling some diarrhea and incontinence. Now, with the continuing proctitis, those problems would only make the transition much harder to bear."

I was choking on my words for one more question.

"What would you do?"

"I'm a doctor. I have to be in control of my life. I would stay with the ileostomy."

In spite of my protestations, I understood the wisdom of what he was saying. I thought back to all the pain I had suffered coming home from the last dilation or from any other test dealing with my rectum.

I was even having a lot of discomfort on a regular basis if I stood on my feet for too long. The thought of enduring diarrhea or incontinence on top of what I was experiencing already was grim. I told him I needed to think about this decision. We made plans to meet again in a week to discuss the issue.

For the next few days, I stayed at home, feeling depressed. I actually wondered if life was worth all of this suffering. I was angry. At whom, for what, I wasn't sure. Was I mad at all the radiation I had been given? That was a question I repeatedly asked myself. But wasn't I cancer free six months since my first diagnosis? So, maybe it was necessary.

I couldn't get beyond the grief I was feeling knowing my body would be altered forever.

Not knowing where to turn, I made an appointment to see Vicki, one of my enterostomal nurses, the following day. She didn't give me any advice, but just listened as I vented my anguish. Then she offered another perspective I had not considered.

"You know Carol, most of the people I see here are grateful for an ostomy. Their lives have been miserable with colitis or other colorectal diseases. An ostomy is enabling them to have a beautiful life. It sounds like this might be the case for you, as well."

What she was saying made a lot of sense.

Vicki continued, "Think about it. On a daily basis, has the ostomy been so hard to live with?"

I played a rerun in my memory of the last six months. Except for the problems caused by the blockages, which were mostly caused by dehydration, I had been saved from all the pain I probably would have had to encounter from diarrhea.

"I guess I have to admit that 98% of the time, the ostomy has not been a problem. I suppose the thought of having it forever is what's making it so hard."

Vicki understood what I meant. "Probably harder for you because you had different expectations, but you know, I think you've been adjusting very well to the idea."

And I had. It wasn't a big deal to me anymore. Even though I thought it was just going to be temporary, I was managing to do everything I wanted to do without letting it interfere with my life.

Vicki went on. "We can equip you with top-of-the-line appliances, and experiment with shapes and sizes. Julie and I will be here to give you all the help that you need if you run into any more roadblocks."

She added, "You might even want to consider joining the Ostomy Association group now and going to their meetings. They're very helpful."

When I left her office, I knew that I had to move on. There was no question what decision I was going to have to make. I wanted to lead the highest quality of life available to me. Some of my vanity would have to go and my ileostomy would have to stay.

When I went back in for a follow-up visit, I told the colorectal surgeon, "I've decided to keep the ileostomy. I'm not so sure how good I'm going to be about it, but I'll do the best job on myself that I'm able to do."

He was sympathetic but obviously relieved.

"You've been courageous so far. I know you will be able to handle this too."

Even though I was still besieged with grief, this vote of confidence helped my outlook. There remained an important question that had been on my mind.

"One thing I have to know. Will having an ostomy shorten my life expectancy?"

He didn't hesitate. "Not a day. Not even a day."

He ended with, "My suggestion is that you finish your treatments and then we will put you on a follow-up schedule. Julie and Vicki will help you with the transition. You'll start to feel better soon. You're going to have a good, long life ahead of you. Embrace it."

So, the reversal of my ileostomy became instead a reversal of my plans to get rid of it. My itinerary had changed and I was changing along with it. I had reached a major crossroad of my journey, choosing a path that would ensure a better way of life for me. It was crucial I made the decision and no one else. That fact alone gave me strength.

Finishing Chemotherapy

By the end of November, I went in to see my oncologist as I approached the last two weeks of my treatments. My decision about choosing not to have the reversal was still too new for me to talk about without tears.

When I told him about it, he looked at me seriously, cracking no jokes this time. He said simply, "I'm sorry."

I told him I thought my colorectal surgeon was disappointed too.

He shook his head and replied, "You know, the hardest thing for a doctor to do is to tell you that the plans you have made together don't look like they are going to work out."

"I know. I think I'm coming around to accepting this, but I'm not there yet."

We reviewed my record for the four dosages of chemo I had just completed. This last month was physically uneventful, which was eventful just for that fact alone. I was now dealing with treatments rather than having them deal with me: Drinking plenty of water, taking medication for nausea when I needed to so that I could eat an adequate diet, balancing activity and resting during the day to accommodate my energy level.

I told him I owed him an apology. I was blaming the chemo for everything that had gone wrong in my body. I realized later dehydration was goofing me up more than anything. Having an ostomy only complicated my situation.

"That's all right," he said, trying to lighten the conversation. "Everyone blames me for everything."

We switched the topic to my fifth treatment. With a new initiative I didn't have before, I threw out a suggestion.

"I always seem to have trouble after my fifth and sixth treatments. Would it be possible to shorten this cycle, and then complete the rest of my chemo after Christmas?"

He listened, thought for a moment or two, and then said, "Actually, I think that's a good idea. In your case, it might do a lot of harm to finish them up. Let's make today your last treatment."

That was what I wanted to hear! Nevertheless, I didn't want to shorten my dosage if that would be better for me to do.

"I'm not finking out too fast, am I?"

He shook his head, smiling, "There's no evidence that finishing these last treatments would make a difference. It's individual. This has been really hard. You should feel very proud of what you have achieved. And your attitude has been superb."

At that moment I felt victorious.

I heartily vowed, "I'll tell you this much. I will never go back to the stress I was under before."

He couldn't let that comment pass. "Wanna bet? All my patients say that. They all want to go out and smell the roses. I bet you a hot fudge malt you will return to being stressed at times because you know why? That's life." We laughed.

I went in for my final zapping of chemotherapy. The nurses who had been there during my worst moments hugged me and said goodbye. I was jubilant, but I made a conscious effort to downplay the fact that I was not coming back. There were too many people sitting there who would be wishing they could say the same.

Freedom

Christmas came once again. It seemed hard to believe that one year prior I was trying to cope with my first diagnosis of malignancy. Here I was, all done with my treatments, feeling better every day. Cancer free and alive!

Our Gang decided against taking a ski trip that year. One of our friends had recently renovated his cabin, and we decided we would spend New Year's Eve up there. As a special treat, he arranged a hayride. I wasn't sure I could make it because my energy level was still low. My appetite was just starting to come back, and I felt more sensitive to cold weather than I had before. As it was, the weather was mild, and we took the trip sitting on some warm comforters and hay. Diehard Minnesotans love the crispness of air in the winter and we were no exception. The bells on the horses jingled all the way, and we were able to stop for a rest at a hunting lodge deep in the forest.

There was one ironic twist. The hunting lodge had no bathroom, only a very, very cold outhouse. Guess who was the only one not worried about using it in an emergency? With an ostomy, you have creative ways of dealing with a wretched bathroom.

On the way back, to enhance his treat of a sleigh ride, our thoughtful friend had taken the time to record some special songs. We all like to sing, so we joined in on our favorite tunes. When Ed Ames came on the tape singing "Try to Remember" it felt like he was singing just to me. Yes, it was deep in December, and I needed to remember the time when grass was green and life was mellow. All the love that was there filled me with gratitude. I had won my freedom and I would do everything in my power to keep it that way.

**Tips for Travelers After Treatments:

- Don't expect to feel better immediately. Chemotherapy keeps on working after you are done with your treatments.
- Practice good nutrition. No diet is magic and can "cure" you of your cancer. Consult your doctor about taking supplements.
- Realize if you've come this far, you're already a winner.
- Drive to your favorite park. Smell the roses. (Or if it's winter, go on a hayride.)
- Buy yourself a hot fudge malt. Spend time with the people you love. Sing. Listen to music. Laugh. Have a glass of wine. Enjoy the sunsets.
- Hug your children. Or your grandchildren. Or any child. Be thankful.

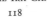

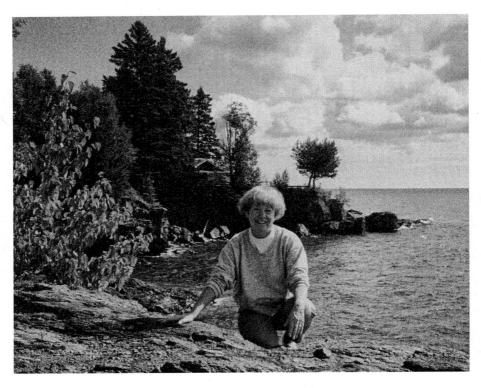

Cancer has no power over the human spirit.

CHAPTER TEN

When the Trip Is Over:
The Lessons Learned
From Surviving Cancer

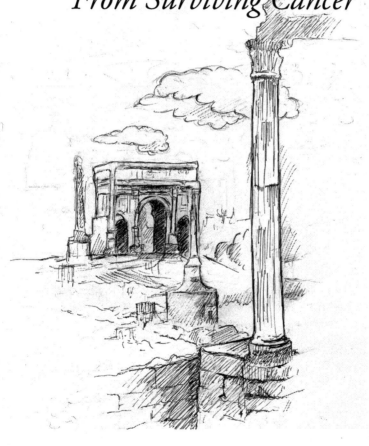

What will I remember about this journey? As our tour of Italy is coming a close, I mentally survey our photographs of Pompeii, the Amalfi Coast, Florence, Venice and Rome. In most of them, Dave and I are posing with our friends in front of world famous tourist attractions, looking like the kind of people you see in advertisements, enjoying ourselves immensely. For the most part, that's true.

Predictably, moments from this trip will someday be preserved in an album. As traveling tends to do, aspects of this journey will influence my view of life. The pictures will be cropped to preserve the best parts of our trip I want to remember. All the inconveniences, discomforts, and problems will fade somewhat with time.

Our final day in Rome begins with picture postcard weather. Everything is according to schedule. By arriving early, we avoid waiting in a long line to visit St. Peter's Cathedral and the Vatican museum. After a two hour tour, we are looking upward to admire Michelangelo's work of art, *The Creation* painted on the ceiling of the Sistine Chapel. God's hand is reaching out to touch the hand of Adam, an electrifying portrayal of the magnificence of life. I am lulled into an illusion of perfection about the artwork we are seeing and about this trip.

Past noon when we leave the Vatican, our guide, Guilia tells us if we hurry through lunch, we can catch another bus to go to the Roman ruins. Finding a nearby cafeteria, I select a bowl of pasta, downing it in record time. I scold myself for doing this. Food needs to be carefully chewed when you have an ileostomy to avoid having it interfere with the passageway. Only after I am through my meal, does it register in my mind that there were quite a few olives and onions mixed in with the dish. I feel as if I am beyond danger at this point, however. In that we go home tomorrow, I don't give it much thought.

We arrive at the ruins and walk up a steep ramp to Capitoline Hill where we have a panoramic view of what remains of the Roman Forum and sur-rounding buildings, broken and amongst the weeds. We have to look beyond the present to appreciate the view. Having a guide helps us to do that. From 509 B.C. when the last king had been overthrown to 44 B.C. when Julius Caesar was assassinated, the Senate became the main governing board of the Roman Republic, answering only to the present Caesar. It was here where debates and discussions took place, where reason would sometimes prevail over chaos and an attempt was made to solve problems by rational means. Although the reality did not always live up to these ideals, this is how the Forum will be remembered.

Today, 2000 years later, we have seen the art of Michelangelo and these famous fragmented monuments of the Forum as the last vestiges of the grandeur of Rome.

We take a picture of this scene facing the ruins posing with smiles on our faces. The photographs are a distortion, however. They do not reflect the truth. By this time I am conscious of the fact I am having mild cramps, a sure sign food is not passing freely through my system. I feel anything but smiley. I realize I might be having the beginnings of a blockage.

It was the same problem that brought me into emergency rooms at least five times in the last two years since I was given an ileostomy. The difference was that Vicki and Julie were not within a phone call away, nor was my colorectal surgeon.

On the way back to our hotel, we decide to rest by stopping at a sidewalk café on a famous street in Rome called Via Veneto, a street known for its chic luxurious hotels and restaurants. By this time, I am trying to drink only liquids and indulge in a cappuccino. We stay there for a while, but the cramping continues, becoming slightly more painful. Dave goes to a nearby store and buys me some grape juice. Even this remedy doesn't work.

The illusion of perfection has vanished. Our wonderful, well-planned trip has changed, at least, for me. I am now facing a potentially dangerous roadblock, which will require all the reasoning I can summon to overcome my fears.

This is one experience that will not be recorded on film.

The Picture That Did Not Get Into the Album

After leaving Via Veneto, Dave and I took a cab back to our hotel room. He watched TV to combat his nervousness as I went into our stark, white hotel bathroom and took out my container of syringes and medical supplies.

I told myself to hold back the panic, live in the present, and tried to remain as rational as I could. I knew I must take immediate action and prioritize what I needed to do, to prevent this from becoming worse. Too much stress could work against me. These last two years have taught me to relax into pain when it occurs. Taking a warm bath helps me to do this, and that's what I did. This time, it didn't work.

In one hour, I was doubled up with cramps by more serious pains, making me feel nauseated. I had some relief in between the spasms and I knew I had to take advantage of these times with more aggressive measures.

"Are you OK in there?" Dave asked me in a voice cloaked with worry.

"I'll be all right" I answered, not sure I meant what I said.

However, I was prepared for this emergency.

Before I left for this trip, Vicki taught me how I could clear a blockage by injecting water into the opening of my stoma and my intestinal passageway. To be honest, the thought that I might have to do this by myself was frightening.

"Are you sure I'm not going to damage my intestine when I do this?" I asked her then.

"You have to be careful," she said, placing a lubricated slender tube in my hand and we practiced the procedure. Attaching a plastic pump full of water to the other end, I proceeded to stick a 16 inch rubber red-orange flexible tube, a quarter inch in diameter, snaking its way into my belly through my stoma, down a space I was never aware existed before.

"Think of yourself like a professional mechanic flushing out a carburetor of a car siphoning out sludge," she suggested.

"That's no good," I replied. "I'm terrible at fixing machines, and that goes double for trying to make repairs on my own body."

"You will be fine," Vicki repeated. "It doesn't hurt, does it?"

"No," I had to admit. "It just looks bad."

That was easy to do when Vicki was watching over me, but now, alone in this bathroom of our Roman hotel, I was on my own. If I failed, I would be forced to rely on foreign medical care, hoping they could speak English better than I could Italian. I had the name and telephone number of an enterostomal nurse in Rome. Dave and I had already marked out the route to the American Hospital about a half hour from our hotel but we were scheduled to go to the airport early the next morning to leave for home. If this turned out to be a full-blown blockage, I might have to end up in an emergency room somewhere in Rome as the pain would become too excruciating to handle it myself. We would then have to stay in Italy and miss our plane should that be the case. I tried to put that thought on the back burner to save myself from boiling over with fear.

I wasn't entirely successful, but after a few tries, I was able to partially unblock the passage, with bits of food coming out with the water. Suddenly, some blood stained water squirted out. I drew a breath in panic. It was only a minor amount, however, and quickly stopped. After twenty more minutes, without another incident, it seemed like I was going to be fine. I actually went a couple of hours without any more pain.

With some worry, Dave and I dressed and went on a minibus to a nearby restaurant for our last night in Rome. I only drank water and clear soup. I was in another picture, uneasily smiling at the camera. My cramps were beginning to return.

We left early to go back to our hotel room. I took another bath and tried to plan my next step. By now, I was beginning to retch. If I took a pain pill, not only would I not be able to keep it down, but also I might end up being dehydrated from losing fluids. The cramps hurt, but not to the extent that they had before. I chose the best course of action I thought I should take. I took a muscle relaxant prescribed to me for this purpose.

Blessedly, I went to sleep, for a few hours.

In the middle of the night, I woke with more pain, vomited, but went back to sleep. By morning I was still mildly uncomfortable but better.

The bus was waiting to take us to the airport. I would have rather stayed in bed, but I also reasoned that in case my efforts had not been successful, at least I would be heading back to the United States, and if the blockage persisted, I could make it back to my home hospital. Enough time had passed, so I could take another muscle relaxant. I fell asleep on the plane, was sick to my stomach in the airport where we changed planes, then slept on the way home to Minnesota. When we came in, I was drinking Gatorade and water to restore my electrolytes and prevent dehydration, looking merely like a tired traveler and not someone who had just averted danger. My daughters, who met us at the airport, knew right away something was wrong, and that the tears in my eyes were from relief, not happiness from completing a memorable trip to Italy.

There is one postscript to this subject. After our trip, I continued to have more blockages and finally was willing to undergo another operation to determine what was causing me so much trouble. The answer was: Plenty. What was discovered was that my body produced a large number of adhesions, which were vying for my attention by causing my colon to sporadically twist. After my colorectal surgeon removed them and created a new stoma for me, a new era of being mostly free of blockages opened up for me.

The Road Back

What happens when life is supposed to become "normal" once again? I wish I could say that once through with all of my treatments, and most of my severe blockage problems solved, that life proceeded on a steady upward swing.

While there was certainly jubilance arriving at this destination, I found new mountains that needed to be conquered before moving on to the next phase: Full recovery.

Every time I go in for a checkup, I have to overcome fears of a recurrence although as each year goes by, I feel less and less insecure. With Stage Three colorectal cancer, five years of good checkups is almost considered a "cure."

The after-effects of radiation proctitis still persist for me and I need to get off my feet every so often to avoid discomfort. I ended up having a crisis during what should have been a normal operation on a benign cyst, but that's another story I've written in a book called *Lifelines*.

Although I never would have chosen such a hard path for myself, I'll have to say that life has been better for me since I've made my way back. I am more appreciative of the ordinary aspects of life that I used to take for granted. It's so wonderful to be able to appreciate the taste of food once again and to have energy to do the things I want to do. When I gaze upon the faces I love, I immediately put them in the album of my mind as souvenirs of the wonderful gift of life.

Cancer is a wretched disease, but it has no power over the human spirit.

Maybe, with time, my memories of my detour with cancer will fade like old photographs. Some of that is good because life goes on. Some of the lessons I've learned, however, I never want to forget for myself and for others because they have made me a more experienced traveler.

Every time I start to get afraid of the future, I think back to that night in Rome and know that whatever the future brings I can handle it. I have a new mission in life to pass on my knowledge to other people, at all stages of cancer, whether they end up with an ostomy or not. My perspective at this juncture is that of a returning traveler returning from the alien territory of cancer to the ordinary concerns of life. I may have taken a long way to get to this point, but oh, it's good to be back home again!

Tips for Travelers in Recovery:

Begin With Realistic Expectations

I found my mind and my emotions did not just immediately stop processing all that has happened to me. I had flashbacks and memories of some of my cancer journey, especially when I was traveling in Rome. Perhaps one trip reminded me of another.

I needed to give myself time to heal. My previous focus on trying to get well changed back to everyday existence. It helped me to think of myself as a vehicle, out of commission for some time. It made sense to give myself a slow, steady start. "Revving" up too fast could stall my engine. I let myself "idle" for a while, preparing for a long, pleasant trip.

Occasional naps were therapeutic. I enrolled in a mild exercise program called T'ai Chi, which not only contributed to a well-exercised body, but also provided me with relaxation while promoting a positive frame of mind. Taking walks, gardening, and moderate exercise were all excellent ways to train myself for a comeback.

I had to remind myself some tiredness was just a part of everyday living and growing older. I told one of my doctors while having an ultrasound, "I don't have as much stamina as I did before."

"Join the club," he said and laughed.

I found that many of my muscles need gradual stretching and strengthening. Eventually, I've found the most comfortable rhythm for my lifestyle, and my endurance slowly increased. As my health improved, my stamina increased. Not to what it was before, but to a new "norm" for me.

Enlist Personal Resources

As I said before, cancer weaves a caring network. The things I took for granted before — good health and being alive — were no longer "givens." It was a fearsome experience, but one that automatically made me a part of a large group. There were medical checkpoints along the way that produced certain amounts of anxiety. As my confidence increased, this lessened in time. Doctors and nurses, as well as cancer survivors, gave me tips that are found on these pages promoting recovery. I find I still need to ask them questions occasionally and enlist others for help. Resources that have been helpful to me are listed at the back of this book.

Above all, I learned to ask my friends and family for help when I needed it. People don't have a crystal ball. They need to know if you want some assistance.

Reduce Unnecessary Stress

My outlook on life has been changed. Once I confronted cancer, I faced my own mortality, and once there, I never forgot it. By living in the present, my life became more spontaneous and exciting than it ever was before.

Specifically, I became more aware of the importance of balancing the demands of stressful situations than I had been before I was diagnosed with cancer. I needed to keep my immune system strong and I knew that too much stress was harmful. My previous level of responsibility, and my reaction to it, needed to be moderated.

After treatment was over, I reevaluated my career. I loved my job, but the stresses were more than I wanted to take on again. I decided to retire from teaching. When I no longer had to go to school, it felt at times like I was playing "hooky." Released from a taxing daily schedule and the demands of my chosen field, every day seemed like a vacation. Time to rest. Time to write. Time to renew valued friendships.

Predictably, the old restlessness of desiring to be a more active person returned. I reminded myself that I might owe my oncologist a hot fudge malt. Stress is a part of life.

Volunteering at a local public library provided the medium for me to use the skills that I had to offer in a different way. I also was able to offer my services for a couple of years working with a dynamic public trainer of the Hennepin County library, and in the process, became a guest columnist for our local newspaper, *The Sun*. Taking classes inspired me to go in a new direction and I became a freelance writer.

Still, I found I ached to be back working with teenagers again. I missed it. To my rescue, my former principal, also a great friend, called.

"Carol, how are you doing?" he asked. When I answered positively, he followed up that question with, "How would you like a job working as a resource person for pregnant teens? As part of a grant, we have an eight hour-a-week position with flexible hours open at one of our alternative schools you could apply for."

I not only was hired for the job. I even had my own office!

At first, I thought I had died and gone to heaven. It was perfect, and I was ecstatic to be back. Then I started to tire. The girls needed more help than I was able to give them for the short time I was there at school. I started worrying, rightly so, that they were being shortchanged. I worked with the school and administration to try to get more funding. The needs were great, the money came through, and then I was able to bow out gracefully, knowing they would benefit from someone who could devote more hours to the job. This time, however, I got to choose when and where I would finally retire from teaching. Being given the right to choose made all the difference.

What opened up for me was a part-time job working at the same library in which I had been volunteering. I found a niche in an environment I loved with an engaging, caring staff and a position that suited me well.

Cultivate an "Attitude"

Being a cancer survivor, there have been so many difficulties to overcome that I was no longer willing to tolerate negative situations that sapped my enjoyment of life. The time to address those problems is now, not some time in the future. I have learned a great deal of problem solving. I find that I am constantly evaluating how I want to spend my time. I've learned the value of having a good day. Connecting with a good friend, exercising, and writing have become top priorities for me. I also have been tending to things in my environment that have been bothering me for years. We hired a neighbor who has a lawn service to plant bushes and trees that would come up on a perennial basis requiring very little work on our part and giving us a beautiful view.

This may sound contradictory, but I also had to learn to slough off unsolvable problems that are really not very important. The challenge here was to know the difference. This was an area needing constant reassessment. It was pointed out to me that the lack of control you sometimes feel as a patient in the course of treatment reverses itself in recovery, as you start to want to control everything. What I needed to cultivate was a new attitude, using my newfound lessons in life to make whatever changes are necessary, if I am able to do so, to improve my quality of life.

Face Unexpected Challenges: The Potholes of Depression

Living in Minnesota, we know about potholes. Winter plays havoc with our highways, and even the best of roads can be pitted with ruts. You can keep driving over them only so long before the constant wear and tear will take a considerable beating on your tires. The same goes for depression and what it does to your immune system.

Probably the cause of most of my down moods was fear. I started to imagine there were insurmountable limitations to my life caused by cancer or having an ostomy. I started to mourn what I would like to do if this had never happened to me. Most of those feelings were in my head and limiting only because I made them that way. When I was having an occasional blockage, a cloud of negativity rained down on me for a few days. Other emotions like self pity, martyrdom, or resentment were there, too, when I least seemed to want them. When I found these feelings were mucking up the road I was on, I worked on not letting them accumulate, so they wouldn't start to permanently ruin the ride.

I find I still have a need to grieve. Whenever that happens, I stop whatever I'm doing and let myself feel anguish for as long as I need to do.

Then, I drive on.

Explore the Private Roads of Sexuality

The important thing to remember when it comes to sex is that intimacy begins in the brain, not in the body. While it's not uncommon for the desire for sex to be diminished during cancer treatments, I'm here to tell you that the good news is that once your body begins to rejuvenate, so does your sex drive. If you once had a healthy sexual appetite, having cancer only temporarily interferes with your capacity to fulfill your needs. Some new changes in your body, like an ostomy, might seem like they would set up roadblocks for sexual pleasure. This is one of those areas I would say, where there is a will, there is a way. With just a little creativity, and perhaps alteration of some sexy undergarments, your body can look better than ever. Coping with changes in appearance fades quickly with a little fantasizing.

There's nothing like good communication to overcome anxiety with any sexual activity, and that's certainly true when combating negative thoughts caused by problems with your health. A good sexual partner can help you to regain your perspective.

If you are a woman, and some changes have occurred after radiation, consult a doctor or a nurse for medical advice and to learn about exercises that may prove to be helpful.

If you are a man, this time, you might really want to ask for directions.

In either case, you can go to an excellent resource, a booklet called "Sexuality and Cancer" from the American Cancer Society. Call toll free 1-800-ACS-2345.

Learn to Live With Other Detours

People who have had ulcerative colitis or a colorectal disease know that having an ostomy is a blessing in restoring a better life than they had before. This is certainly true in my case, as opposed to struggling with the all the problems I would have without help.

After cancer, the needs of my body changed, and new dietary concerns have become part of my daily life. I learned that I was the best moderator of my own health. Instead of following past routines, I need to check to see if what I am doing is healthy for me or consult someone knowledgeable in nutrition for advice.

Usually, the ostomy that I have now has come to be a non-issue in my life as far as preventing me from doing anything I want to do. It is clean, efficient, and safe. After my trip to Rome, I knew I could travel anywhere I wanted to with confidence, knowing there were enterostomal nurses and services around the world for me to access.

I always need to be prepared for emergencies: plenty of water, extra supplies, and medication if things are not going smoothly for me. I have had to learn the hard way that I have to be careful about what I eat and to carefully chew my food. There is a gem of a book called, Yes, We Can! It is listed in the resource section after this chapter and is full of good suggestions.

At times, I've become quite smug about the fact that I do not have to face the same kind of emergencies other travelers might encounter. I never will have to worry about bathroom cramps on a long bus ride. I have a distinct advantage if we are traveling in a rural area abroad, and there is just a hole in the ground toilet for tourists to use.

Sometimes, I feel that the old way of "doing business" is perfectly barbaric!

Of course, this is said now with a lot of adjusting on my part.

The lesson I've learned from having an ostomy is that it's not what is done to you that produces such a difference, but what you make of it that counts. Every time I start to feel bad about having an ostomy, and believe me, this still is something I have to work on, I remind myself of the high quality of life I am living now and how thankful that I am living at a time when this has become easier than it was before because of new disposable appliances and 100% effective deodorizers.

Arrivederci

Having cancer increased my appreciation for friends and loved ones. They were my lifelines when I needed them most, and there is a sense of gratitude I have for them I will never lose. However, there is another huge source of emotional support that may not be quite so apparent.

When I was battling cancer, my calendar was dotted with appointments to see doctors and the nurses who were doing everything they could to keep me well. When it was no longer necessary for me to see them on a regular basis, I expected to feel elated. Instead, the month following my last appointment, I found myself oddly sad. I was so thankful that the cancer seemed to be gone, and my trek with cancer was hopefully over, but now, I was feeling scared and uneasy. I couldn't quite figure this out. I am not a dependent person, and I certainly "have a life." What was bothering me? To figure this out, I enlisted the help of an insightful psychologist at the hospital.

She helped me see that the people I was leaving were the ones who guided me to safety and who were with me down the dark roads when the going was really rough. No way did I want to return to the difficulties I had before, but I would always be grateful they were there. I was lost, and I was so glad they came along when they did. It was time for me to move on, but I know where to look if I ever need help again.

So my story, as well as my trip to Italy, will become part of my past.

I am still having trouble with the concept that the cancer I experienced was a "gift", but I certainly am aware that many gifts have come to me because of the experience. The lessons I have learned from having cancer are simply:

• Celebrate life.
• Keep my time well balanced with the demands of work and the other aspects of my life that are important to me.
• Seek the most positive solutions to my problems.
• Don't get stuck in negative ruts.
• Give support to others as a way to thank the people who have helped me along the way.

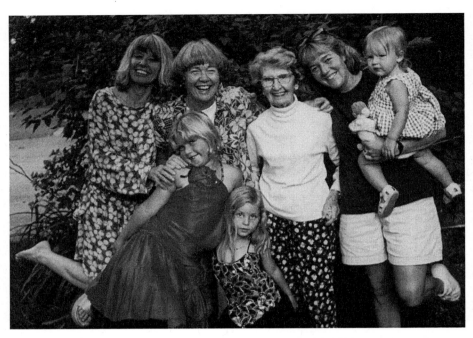

Meg, Courtney, me, Aisha (Meg's granddaughter), Jean, Tami, and daughter Kailey (born after I was done with all my treatments)

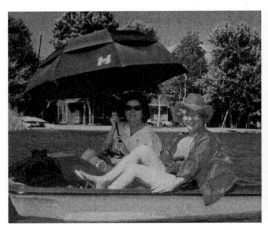

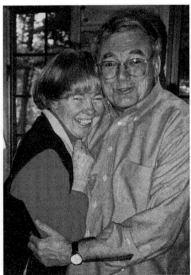

My pal Marilyn and me at the lake. Dave and I know how much we have to be thankful for.

CHAPTER ELEVEN

Moving On

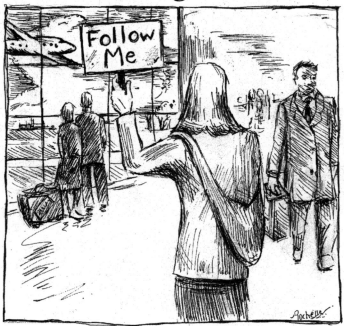

After I recovered from my ordeals, I realized that I wanted to pass on what I had learned from my experiences. My journey had ended but now I wanted to prevent or diminish the devastating after-effects of colorectal disease for other people. What surfaced was a deep commitment on my part to help others in my predicament just as others had helped me. This is a common reaction for people who have lived through a hard time in their lives. According to psychiatrist, Alfred Adler, our emotional well-being and sense of worth is significantly shaped by how much we make an effective contribution to society.

Support groups give us this opportunity. By helping others, we help ourselves.

Joining A Grass-Roots Support Group: ACE

In 1999, I heard about a grass-roots colorectal cancer support group. Cindy Iverson, developmental director of the Colon and Rectal Foundation, along with others, was establishing Advocates for Colorectal Education (ACE). I called one of the members, and was lucky to link up with Ruth Edstrom, who was the editor of their newsletter. She was caring, vivacious, and competent. I'll never forget that first meeting with Ruth. We became immediate and long-lasting friends. She asked me if I wanted to help her with their newsletter, "The Advocate." Ruth is an inspiration to all who know her. Her cancer had spread to her liver and metastasized but in her words, Ruth said:

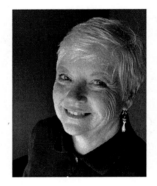

Ruth Edstrom

"I believed that for every type and severity of cancer, there were some who survived. And why shouldn't I be one of them? At that time, Katie Couric was getting her colonoscopy done on nationwide television. And Charles Schultz, the creator of the Peanuts cartoon series, died from colon cancer. So public awareness of the disease was high, and statistics were everywhere." Ruth tried not to take the statistics personally, endured surgery and some harsh side effects. Today she is still cancer-free. She has made it her mission to spread this message: *"Get screened. It could save your life."*

Besides the newsletter, ACE made visitations, gave speeches and attended legislative activities. Barney Palmer was the first president and Jane Nielsen took the job over once he left for Florida. Both Jane and Ruth helped me to edit and self-publish this first book in 2003. Julie Weaver, a leading actress in "How to Talk Minnesotan" headed our speakers' group and Paul Leland was our treasurer. Out of this group emerged Mary Bakke, who facilitated a colorectal support group at North Memorial Hospital. (See article on page 136.) At that time, they were the only support group dedicated to colorectal cancer in the Twin Cities. Mary had created beautiful, iridescent bracelets, which she called, "Buddy Bracelets" to give people to remind them to have a colonoscopy. On March 5th, 2005, Mary was honored as a Blue Cross Blue Shield, "Minnesota Champion of Health." Her Buddy

Bracelet, in a more sporty form, became used by advocates across the country.

ACE participated in television spots and phone banks gaining media atttention. In 2005, Cindy Iverson, as the new director for the Minnesota Colon and Rectal Foundation, along with the Cancer Research and Prevention Foundation (CPRF) arranged to have the "Colossal Colon" come to Minneapolis.

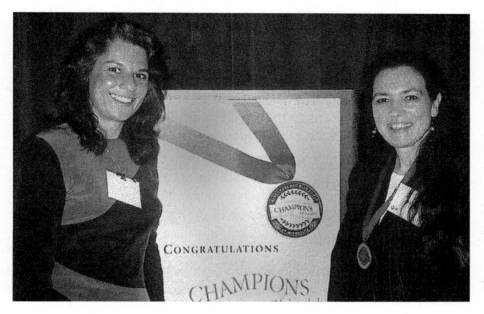

Cindy Iverson and Mary Bakke at the Blue Cross Blue Shield Award ceremony.

The North Memorial Group-A Self-Help Support Group

As Mary Bakke once said, "There are times in our lives when we need the support of others to get us through tough ordeals. It could be our family, friends or neighbors, or a support group. The emotional, spiritual, and physical support is fulfilling and uplifting." Mary and Jane VanDuessen-Morrison started facilitating the North Memorial Colorectal Support Group which has served as a valuable resource for patients who have been diagnosed with colorectal cancer. It did not matter whether patients had currently undergone treatment or in the past. Any colorectal cancer survivor and their support person and family were welcome to attend. They did not have to be a patient of North Memorial to attend this group. People in this group had access to two dynamic facilitators; Mary, a colon cancer survivor and Jane, a Professor of Nursing who was also an oncology nurse.

They have a set-up that works: A light dinner is served and meetings consist of either a speaker who presents information on a topic that is relevant to cancer patients and their supporters, or they have an open discussion night. Even if there is a speaker there is always time at the beginning of the meeting where people can update the group on how they are coping with side effects and treatments, simply telling their story or whatever they feel like sharing. This group provides cancer survivors and their families a safe place to come and share their stories about the situation they are facing. They share as much or as little as they want to about their individual situations and ask questions from their medical facilitator, receiving hugs from each other, applauding each other when good news is received, or comforting each other when things are not going as well, and even laughing together if the time is right. They know they are a part of a group of people that all share a special and common bond because they have traveled the same road, perhaps with some different turns along the way. They understand and share each other's frustrations and feelings.

The group is still thriving. Sue Norby, describes it as "a group so unique and special that many of us feel like we are brothers and sisters in the battle against cancer. There is no other place where we can have such openness and honesty with other people like this group. They help you to manage your life during this emotional roller coaster you're riding. Where else can you go and talk about colonoscopies while you are eating dinner and think nothing of it? Support groups like this one and others like the St. Paul and Minneapolis ostomy chapters are much more than just support groups – it's a group of friends who care deeply about one another and share in the joys and sorrows of each and every person's cancer journey."

Forming a New Self-Help Support Group

Matt Rudberg and Kim Ness contacted me recently wanting to talk to me about their new support group, the Colon, Anal, Rectal Support group (CARS). When I met with Matt I tried to give him an overview about some of the support groups I knew for colorectal cancer in the Minneapolis area. Today, there is a growing network in the Metro area and nationally for survivors and their families. Matt asked an important question: "How do you start?" On the way home, I thought that this question should be in this book, so I made some notes:

• Assessment is a key issue. Take people where they are and what they are facing. Newly diagnosed? Into treatments? Recovery?
• Let members talk, and listen to their needs.
• Establish trust and confidentiality.
• Give members the freedom to express themselves honestly.
• Bring in experts and other patients who been on this journey.
• Encourage family members and friends to attend your meetings.
• Most of all, care.

National Organizations: CCC and GYRIG

By 2005, ACE had evolved into supporting a national group founded by Kristin Tabor, the Colon Cancer Coalition. Cindy Iverson became its director. According to Kristin, this coalition began as a dream for her sister Susie Lindquist Mjelde, who succumbed to the disease in August of 2002 at the age of 46. "Get Your Rear In Gear" was Susie's own slogan and it became a message telling people to take charge of their own lives by getting screened. Over the years, Kristin has volunteered and raised thousands of dollars for other charitable organizations. To learn more, go to getyourrearingear.com

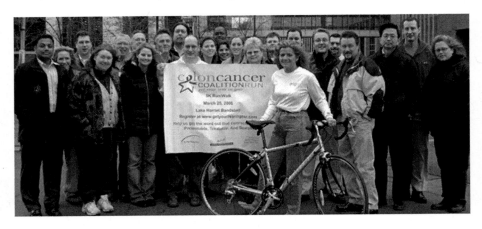

Kristin Tabor, founder of the Get Your Rear in Gear Run

The mission of the Colorectal Cancer Coalition is:
- Partnering with local and national corporations, media, and foundations, survivors, and their families and friends to raise awareness for colon cancer by establishing a colon cancer run and/or an existing run in every state.
- To assist local organizers in directing funds raised at these events to the best programs to fulfill the mission.

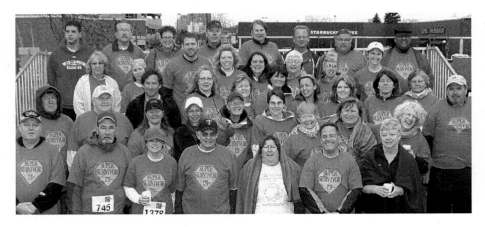

Survivors of colorectal cancer from the 2009 Get Your Rear in Gear Run.
Mary Bakke is in the center fourth row, Brenda is in the second row between
Julie Weaver and me, and Ruth Edstrom is at the end of the first row.

UOAA, The United Ostomy Association of America and OAMA

At a national level, UOAA is a network for bowel and urinary diversion support groups in the United States. Its goal is to provide a nonprofit association that will serve to unify and strengthen its member support groups, which are organized for the benefit of people who have, or will have intestinal or urinary diversions and their caregivers. Go to www.uoaa.org.

I finally had to accept the fact that having an ostomy was going to be a permanent part of my life for me. I realized that I needed more information and support to make this adjustment as good as I could. Vicki and Julie encouraged me to join the Minneapolis chapter of the UOAA. The first time I attended their meeting, I met the President, Karen Tourdot, the president elect, Mike Carlson, and his sister Marilyn who was also a Board member. "Remarkable people" I remember thinking. The meeting was fun! Not dreary and depressing. And then I met someone who was going to have a profound effect on my life: Brenda Elsagher.

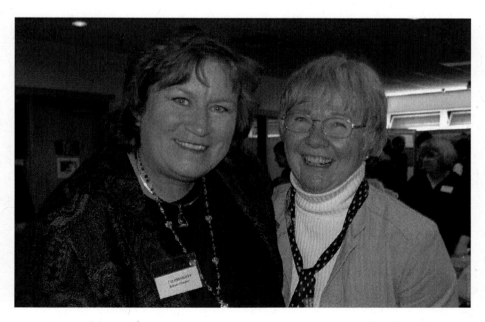

Brenda Elsagher and me.

When I first listened to Brenda speak, I thought, "Who is this woman?" She could be outrageous while making the crowd feel better about their sorrows, funny when talking about a serious matter, a teacher of some extraordinarily complex subjects, teasing while being compassionate. We clicked. We got to know each other better and I felt less afraid to let others know about my surgeries, in particular, my ileostomy. Brenda explained that it wasn't so bad having an ostomy; it was just hard to find shoes to match her bag!

Our friendship grew and soon I found out how persuasive she could be: she talked me into taking on my first presidency of our Minneapolis group. That year, everything went wrong. Our national ostomy group was going through reorganization. The building we were holding our local meetings in was sold. Dues for everyone were in flux. But we came through, and then we found out we were both writing a book. Hers was humorous, *If the Battle is Over, Why Am I Still in Uniform?"* and I went into the first printing of this book. Brenda came out with a new book in 2006, *I'd Like to Buy A Bowel, Please.* Hunter House, a national company, published my second book, *Positive Options for Colorectal Cancer.* We supported each other, and when, in 2007, I had a medical crisis that put me in a coma and a hospital stay of 80 days, who should walk in wearing a floppy hat, but Brenda! I was at my lowest and I didn't think anyone could make me smile, but she did.

Brenda has recently written another book, called *Bed Pan Banter.* She included my stories in both books. I wrote about her in my two books. We decided last year to do a duet, or I should say she talked me into it, and we became co-presidents of OAMA, our Ostomy Association of the Minneapolis Area. We followed that year up with presenting a workshop on "How to Have Fun Meetings" at the 2009 national Ostomy convention in New Orleans. Her website says it all: "Brenda Brings Laughter with a Message." She has become a national comedian and received the "Advocacy to Action Award" of 2009 from the Colon Cancer Coalition. I've seen her take a crowd and turn them into fun-loving people with just an introduction. Her books are fun to read, informative and therapeutic, no matter what happens to be troubling you at the time, ostomy or no ostomy. She is a delightful writer, a good person, and someone that I know I will always call my friend. To get to her website, go to Brenda@livingandlaughing.com.

Legislative Support Groups-C3

When I was first diagnosed with cancer, I wanted to connect with someone who had traveled the same road I was about to travel. I needed to talk to someone – fast. I found an online patient support group founded by Kate Murphy. I mostly followed the conversation of other people who were part of a chat group, but this was so much more important than just chat. I was given helpful information and emotional courage. In 2008, I was awarded the C3 Breaking Boundaries Award and asked to come to Washington to lobby for colorectal cancer. I met Kate Murphy for the first time, who was also an award winner, and other dynamic participants. I learned that the C3 Colorectal Cancer Coalition is a non-profit, nonpartisan advocacy organization that fights colorectal cancer through research, empowerment and access. According to their 2009 website, this organization pushes for research to improve screening, diagnosis, and treatment of colorectal cancer; for policy decisions that make the most effective colorectal cancer prevention and treatment available to all; and for increased awareness that colorectal cancer is preventable, treatable, and beatable. Nationally headquartered near Washington D.C., C3 supports the work of research and grassroots advocates throughout the United States.

Dave and I became advocates for the "Cover Your Butt" campaign www.CoverYourButt.org which supports legislation to guarantee coverage for nearly every American that should be screened: those belonging to the poor and underserved, the elderly and those with private insurance.

Colorectal Cancer Coalition
1414 Prince Street, Suite 204
Alexandria, VA 22314
Toll-free answer line: 1-877-427-2111
Email: info@fightcolorectalcancer.org

The American Cancer Society-Relay for Life

The American Cancer Society is legend for their services for cancer patients and their families. Once a year, volunteers from all walks of life gather in communities to celebrate survivors and in remembrance of loved ones who've lost their lives to cancer. The American Cancer Society has done a wonderful job to raise awareness not only of breast cancer, but colorectal cancer as well. As a national organization, they have clout to exert influence on all levels of government advocating for stronger policies to enact legislation that will save lives and conquer cancer. Go to their website: www.relayforlife.org

It's important to remember that people facing cancer have to determine what they need for support. We can reach out, however, and let them know what resources are out there for them. If you are starting a support group, you need dynamic leaders to initiate the process such as Cindy Iverson, Kristin Tabor, Mary Bakke, and Jane VanDuessen-Morrison. You also need enthusiastic members to turn the group into a place where its members will be met with acceptance and caring concern, such as Ruth Edstrom, Sue Norby, and Brenda Elsagher.

**Tips for Joining a Support Group:

Is this the right kind of group for you?

Would you be more comfortable using an online support group?

Does the group have a clear focus? Are meetings well run?

What is going to be asked of you as a member?

Are your feelings well-received? Do people listen to new ideas?

Is there a sense of camaraderie?

**Tips for Starting a Support Group

Do any already exist that would address your concerns?

Are there other organizations that the group could align with?

Visit and talk with other support group leaders

Is there funding available?

How will you publicize information about the group?

Advocates

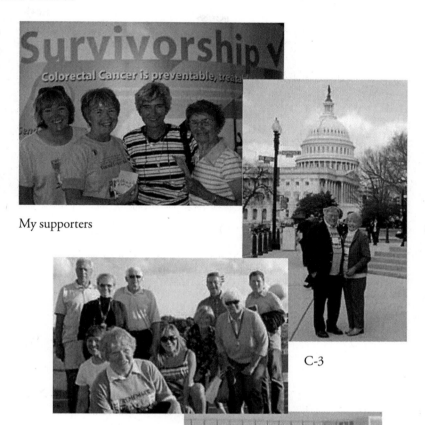

My supporters

C-3

Relay for Life

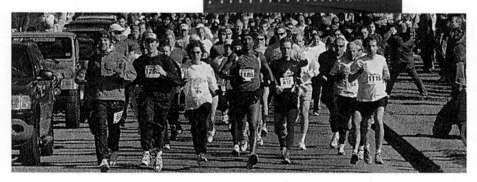

Get Your Rear In Gear!

Bibliography

ITALIAN REFERENCES

Rick Steve's Italy, Amazon.com 2009

Frommer's 2009 Italy, Amazon.com 2009

Tanaka, Shelly, *The Buried City of Pompeii: What It Was Like When Vesuvius Exploded,* Madison Books, 1997

Dryansky, G.Y., "We'll always have Amalfi," *Conde Nast Traveler,* New York, May 1996

"Beyond Naples," *Rick Steve's Travel News* www.ricksteves.com

King, Ross, *Brunelleschi's Dome — How a Renaissance Genius Reinvented Architecture,* Penguin Books 2000

Gates of Paradise www.gracecathedral.org/church/crypt/cry19960703.shtml

History and Interpretation of Gladiatorial Games; Roman gladiators; roman history; roman civilization (http//abacus.bates.edu/~mimber/Rciv/gladiator.htm)

Roman Culture: www.campus.northpark.edu/historyt//WebChron/Mediterranean/Gladiators. htmal

ARTICLES

"Colon Cancer, The Secret Cancer," *Living Smarter,* PO Box 9310 Mpls, MN. Spring, 1999

Broderick, Richard. "The Last Taboo," published by the University of Minnesota Alumni Association at McNamara Alumni Center, 200 Oak Street SE, Suite 200, Minneapolis, MN. 55455-2040, September-October 2001

PAMPHLETS

Patient brochures from Colon and Rectal Associates, Ltd.

Myths and Facts About Colorectal Cancers — what you need to know Pazdur, M.D.,Richard and Royce, M.D., Melanie. PRR,Inc., publishers of ONCOLOGY, 17 Prospect Street, Huntington, NY,11743, July 2007

National Health Information Center
816-932-8453 (Voice)
800-227-2345 (Toll free)

BOOKS

Colon and Rectal Cancer: A Comprehensive Guide for Patients & Families, Johnston, Lorraine, Patient-Centered Guides, a subsidiary of O'Reilly & Associates, Inc., January 2000

If The Battle Is Over, Why Am I Still In Uniform? Humor as a Survival Tactic to Combat Cancer, I'd Like To Buy a Bowel, Please and *Bedpan Banter,* Elsagher, Brenda. Contact Amazon.com or www.brendabringsjoy.com

Positive Options for Colorectal Cancer, Larson, Carol, Hunter House, 2005 Contact Amazon.com and *Lifelines* contact clarsoneditor.com

Yes We Can! Advice on Traveling With an Ostomy and Tips for Everyday Living, Kupfer, Barbara; Foley-Bolch, Kathy; Kasouf, Michelle Fallon; Sweeney, MD, W. Brian; Chandler House Press Books, 2000

MAGAZINES

Coping, P.O. Box 682268, Franklin, TN 37068

Cure, Sammons Cancer Center, Suite 4802, Dallas TX 75246-9930

Stressfree Living, 14070 Commerce Ave. Suite 200, Prior Lake, MN. 55372

The Phoenix, P.O. Box 3605, Mission Vejo, CA 92690 www.uoaa.org

ONLINE RESOURCES

Association of Cancer Online Resources, www.acor.org

Colon Cancer Alliance, ACOR/CCA www.ccalliance.org

American Society of Colon and Rectal Surgeons www.fascrs.org

American Gastroenterological Association www.gastro.org

American Cancer Society: Colon and Rectum Cancer Resource Center
www.3cancer.org

National Cancer Institute www.cancer.gov

Mayo Foundation for Medical Education and Research MFMER:
www.mayo.edu MedicineNet.com

Colon and Rectal Cancer: A Patient Centered Guide for Colon and Rectal
Cancer www.patientcenters.com

Alternative Cancer Therapies FAQ- Frequently Asked Questions
www.curezone.com/diseases/cancer/faq.htm

Questionable Cancer Therapies, Stephen Barrett, M.D. Victor Herbert,
M.D.J.D. www.quckwatch.com.

COLORECTAL CANCER ORGANIZATIONS

American Cancer Society National Office
599 Clifton Road NE
Atlanta, GA 30329-4251
Phone: (800) ACS-2345

Colon Cancer Alliance, ACOR/CCA
175 Ninth Avenue
New York, NY 10011

Cancer Hot Line Number 1-800-433-0464

THE COLON CANCER COALITION

The Coalition's primary areas of focus are:

• Expanding the existing Get Your Rear in Gear 5K walk/run race and creating new Get Your Rear in Gear events to help increase awareness and funding.

• Providing information about colorectal cancer screening throughout the state and especially in the workplace setting.

• Investing in model programs that will help those underinsured or noninsured to receive colorectal cancer screening.

• Establishing support groups and other support networks for those individuals and families receiving a diagnosis of colorectal cancer.

Colon Cancer Coalition
8009 34th Ave., Suite 360
Bloomington, MN 55425
www.getyourrearingear.com

Please contact the Colon Cancer Coalition for more information.

About the Author

Carol Larson has written a personal, practical, and heartfelt account of her battle with colorectal cancer that could be meaningful to anyone who is facing adversity. With occasional humor, and a positive approach, Carol has uniquely chronicled each phase of her story into a unique format of a guidebook, using images from a recent trip to Italy. Written from her perspective of being a cancer survivor, *When the Trip Changes* has a powerful message to deliver: That cancer can be overcome and despite the difficulties, a new path of life can emerge richer from the experience.

Ms. Larson was a teacher in the St. Louis Park school system, Minnesota, for 24 years, and was a guest columnist for the *Sun* newspaper for two years. Two of her articles, "The Road Back" and "Lessons Learned from Having Cancer" have appeared in the national magazine, *Coping With Cancer*. Her article, "The Road to Recovery" appeared in *Stressfree* magazine. Carol was co-editor for the ACE newsletter, and President of the Minneapolis Ostomy chapter. In 2008, she was named one of the "Women Who Have Broken Barriers for Colorectal Cancer" by the national Colorectal Cancer Coalition and is the mother of three daughters. Carol resides in Minnetonka, Minnesota with her husband, Dave Larson.

To obtain her other books, *Positive Options for Colorectal Cancer* and *Lifelines,* contact Amazon.com.

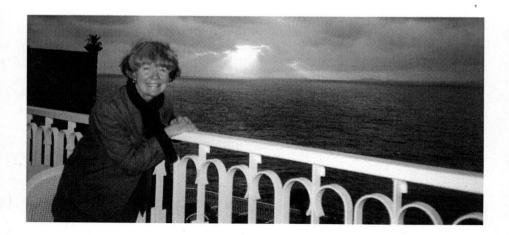